Lecture Notes in Medical Informatics

Edited by D. A. B. Lindberg and P. L. Reichertz

14

F. Wingert

Medical Informatics

An Introduction

Springer-Verlag
Berlin Heidelberg New York 1981

Author

F. Wingert
Westfälische Wilhelms-Universität
Institut für Medizinische Informatik und Biomathematik
Hüfferstr. 75, 4400 Münster, Germany

Exclusively authorized English translation of the original German edition MEDIZINISCHE INFORMATIK published in the series "Leitfäden der angewandten Informatik" edited by L. Richter and W. Stucky © B.G. Teubner, Stuttgart 1979.

ISBN-13: 978-3-642-87463-5 e-ISBN-13: 978-3-642-87461-1
DOI: 10.1007/978-3-642-87461-1

Library of Congress Cataloging in Publication Data
Wingert, F. (Friedrich), 1939– Medical informatics.
(Lecture notes in medical informatics; 14) Translation of: Medizinische Informatik.
Bibliography: p. Includes index. 1. Medicine--Data processing. I. Title. II. Series. [DNLM:
1. Computers. 2. Information retrieval systems. 3. Medicine. WI LE334N v. 14 / W 26.5
W 769m] R858.W5913. 610'.28'5. 81-16561 ISBN 0-387-10870-X AACR2

Softcover reprint of the hardcover 1st edition 1981

2145/3140-543210

Preface to the English Edition

With the exception of some additions in Section 3.1 and minor changes, the English edition of the "Medizinische Informatik" is a translation of the German edition.

Because there is frequently no one-to-one correspondence between the German and the English terminology, misinterpretations are possible. I have tried to avoid this situation as far as possible. The main problem remains within the academic setting. In recent years, the term **informatics** has become popular in Europe, but is widely unknown in the United States. The field covers mostly what is understood as **computer science** and **information science**. The corresponding term **medical informatics**, now used in the name of international societies such as the "International Medical Informatics Association", covers "medical computer science", "medical information science", as well as "biomedical engineering" and has no definite boundary to "biomathematics".

The book has not been translated on a professional basis in order to keep my own style, although there has been assistance by Dr. S. Raymond, for which I am very grateful.

Dipl.-Phys. N. Osada has been of great help both by proof-reading and by excellent support during preparation of the camera-ready manuscript.

Further valuable advice has been given by: A.W. Pratt, M.D.; M. Ebstein, Ph.D.; M. Pacak, Ph.D.; G.S. Dunham; L.D. Nadel, Ph.D.; P.O. Miller.

44 Münster, May 1981 F. Wingert

Preface

This book is an attempt to systematically present problems and methods in a field, which is at present described mainly by the development and application of computer-based systems to aid in the solution of medical problems. Medical informatics lacks a prerequisite of the classical definition of a scientific discipline, namely an independent methodology. This stems from the fact that medical phenomena cannot completely be explained by means of a single science, because biological problems are multi-dimensional in nature.

This situation, together with the broad spectrum of support required for the solution of medical problems, results in a diffuse concept of the field. Thus, it is difficult for the student to obtain a systematic survey of the whole field.

Two further aspects also necessitate a systematic survey:

- It is increasingly necessary to integrate medical informatics into medical knowledge, in order that physicians be aware of the current efforts in the field and eventually contribute to its development.
- The view is gradually gaining in popularity that students of informatics should be made familiar with the opportunities of their discipline as early as possible, which are mainly located in application areas. This systematic survey is intended to acquire and interest the students in practical medical applications and is especially important, because the principles of medical informatics are in parts substantially different from those of other information processing applications.

Experience has indicated that cooperation between physicians and information scientists is often burdened by serious communication problems. Frequently, each professional does not appreciate the opportunities and needs of the "complementary" discipline. Not only does each field have its own technical vocabulary, but in many instances identical terms bear entirely different meanings.

Cooperation between physicians and information scientists is desirable, not only for scientific but also for financial reasons. The budget of a medical school absorbes about 50% of the total budget of a university;

the costs for acquisition and operation of electronic data processing equipment have increased steadily for years, in spite of the significant decrease in hardware costs through the use both of large and small computer systems in many departments. These facts define the necessity for financial economy in medical informatics.

The methods presented here reflect the subjective interests of the author. With increasing consolidation of the discipline during the next few years, efforts to define and systematize the domain are expected to increase. I hope this book will contribute to this development.

The mathematical sections may be omitted by the reader who desires to obtain an understanding of the most important principles. The glossary in Chapter 10 may help in comprehending the whole: it contains the definition of important terms not defined elsewhere in the text.

I gratefully acknowledge the support of many colleagues:

Dr. E. Glowatzki, Prof. Dr. H.-J. Kretschmann, Dipl.-Math. E. Hultsch, Dipl.-Phys. N. Osada, and Prof. Dr. St. Braun who have contributed by proof-reading and by valuable advice. M. v. Os has drawn the figures. I thank H.-D. Siepmann for typing the manuscript.

44 Münster, July 1979 F. Wingert

Contents

1. Information Processing in Medicine

1.1 Introduction

Information processing (i.e., data acquisition, error control, interpretation, and inference) is a fundamental process of medicine as old as medicine itself. Hence, the development of a special discipline for information processing in medicine may at first seem paradoxical, but it has been initiated by far-reaching changes inside and outside the medical profession.

> **Inside** the medical profession, advanced technology has produced new data (e.g., diagnostic data in nuclear medicine and prenatal care); it has also speeded up data production, leading indirectly to new data, which could not be effectively produced before due to limited technology (e.g., multichannel autoanalyzer in the clinical laboratory). The increase in the number and in the degree of differentiation of the techniques for examination and care have increased the specialization in medicine. This all resulted in a significant increase in the number and types of known disturbances of health, which may be recognized and treated. The development of **preventive medicine** has reduced the incidences of previously life-threatening diseases such as tuberculosis. But greater life expectation leads to the appearance of geriatric diseases almost unknown in the past.
>
> In addition, developments **outside** the medical profession influence the spectrum and the significance of diseases. The growing mobility of the population has extended the ranges of formerly localized communicable diseases. For example, tropical diseases are no longer a rarity in Central Europe.

Shifts in the demand and in the need for medical services have consequences for medicine. Those who demand medical services can be classified into (1) the group that needs medical services and (2) the group that does not need medical services, but health information and education. Public health services seek to identify among those not voluntarily demanding medical services the ones who really need medical care.

Formerly, medicine emphasized individual **patient care**. This highly specialized area of diagnosis and therapy requires the most expensive medical services. Modern insurance systems have practically abolished the direct payment for medical services, which in the past has regulated the demand. With the growing concern for health this has caused a shift among the different groups of the population, marked by a steadily increasing proportion of the population demanding services. Traditional medical care is not readily adapted to this process. In practice, this means that physicians have to invest their time in the wrong place. Instead of concentrating on diagnosis and therapy of sick people, physicians become preoccupied with the separation of the sick from the healthy.

Public health organizations can meet the steadily changing demands only if institutions are established, which take into account the needs of the different groups. These institutions have to apply different means when limited resources are to be used optimally. Optimization requires that tasks are transferred from physicians to paramedical personnel. We must also determine whether and how far automated procedures can be applied. Shifts between the above-mentioned groups of the population require extensive communication between institutions serving them.

Medicine is action-oriented: evaluation and action are in a continuous interaction, and we are interested only in information that influences action. In many areas, recognition of the relations between data, as well as their classification and interpretation, have not kept pace with the increased amount of data; as a result, physicians often face a decreasing amount of information from an increasing amount of data.

In **public health policy** a similar phenomenon can be observed. Hospital planning is based on indices such as number of beds for a medical specialty per 1,000 people. But we know very little about how such indices should be set.

To an increasing extent, mathematical modelling is employed in planning. For example, the number of beds in a teaching hospital is calculated from such parameters as the number of patients per student and the percentage of patients suitable for teaching. These plans, derived from mathematical models, seem to result in well-substantiated data if examined superficially. But they lose their value rapidly when parameters are manipulated to obtain a predetermined result, as is the case when the parameters are iterated until the desired number of beds results.

It is, therefore, important to abolish the imbalance between the precision of the methods and the manipulation of the parameters. This must be achieved by the definition of goals and by considering the influence of parameters on the attainability of the goals. We must recognize the danger of interpreting the results of mathematical methods as exact just because the method is exact. Problems involved in selecting appropriate methods and defining appropriate parameters are often neglected. As long as operational definitions in medicine are lacking, we can expect that they will be replaced by definitions oriented towards non-medical (e.g., political or financial) objectives.

Information theory affords important support for these tasks. SHANNON and WIENER, during and after the second world war, elucidated **information** as a fundamental concept, like energy, made it accessible to mathematical treatment, and provided a prerequisite for the development of computer methods.

Methodological foundations have to be created if technologic and scientific developments are to be used to the necessary extent. The methods of informatics have to be harmonized with the possibilities and the needs of medicine. This will require developments in informatics, and even more in medicine, based on close cooperation between information scientists and physicians. No single medical specialty can take over this task. Medical informatics is the new discipline that will do so.

1.2 Overlap With Other Disciplines

"Information processing" in medicine has no well-defined boundaries. There is such a great need for data processing methods, and the complexity of the problem is such that borrowing is necessary from many other disciplines.

The most important ones are:

- mathematics
    - pure mathematics
        - analysis
        - logic
        - probability theory
        - decision theory
    - applied mathematics
    - numerical mathematics
    - statistics
- informatics
    - computer science
    - information science
    - artificial intelligence
- operations research
- information and documentation
    - bibliography
- computational linguistics
- engineering.

Therefore, it is easy to understand that different scientists have different interests depending on their scientific background and training. At present, there is no systematized classification of tasks or methods in medical informatics. The terms used depend on claims of intellectual authorship of information processing in medicine: biomathematics, medical statistics, medical informatics, medical information processing, medical documentation, and so on.

The strength of the mathematically oriented sciences, including informatics, consists of the abstraction of a specific problem to such a level that one can start from axioms, apply explicit logical inferences in a consistent system, and reach general solutions. In most cases, the effectiveness of this approach cannot be questioned. If there is a general solution for a specific problem, then it is only necessary to make minor adaptations to the special situation. This may save enormous investment in obtaining a particular solution. But the level of abstraction may be such that a general solution is of no help at all in a special situation. There are many examples of problems in medicine arising from the peculiarities of a given situation and inhibiting the construction of an elegant "generalized" solution.

In a situation where a patient has one of two possible diseases, and the therapy for one disease implies an adverse reaction to the course of the other disease, even the best computer-assisted diagnosis is of no help, because the only outcome of such a diagnosis is a statement about populations and not about observation units (the probability of a diagnosis for a patient is a statement about a population, i.e., statistics relates to a population of patients and not to a specific patient).

In modern informatics there is a tendency towards higher abstraction, which sometimes gives the impression that it shall be proved that, in spite of the separation from mathematics, informatics still belongs to the "exact" sciences. But in many areas outside informatics the immediate needs are so heavy that solutions have to be sought before the problem can be defined well enough to satisfy theoretic requirements of informatics.

It is almost generally accepted that there has to be a discipline in medicine with special responsibility for information processing. Its denotation is of minor importance, but some main fields and differentiations seem to emerge:

- **Biomathematics** as the union of all mathematical methods in biology and especially in medicine.
- **Medical information processing** as superimposed concept including all methods for acquisition, control, processing, and interpretation of information. In this sense, medical diagnostic processes belong to medical information processing.

- **Medical informatics** as the union of all methods of informatics in medicine including the preparation of medical data required for the application of these methods.

In public health, epidemiology and planning of health systems are especially important. Some authors rank the respective methods with medical informatics, but they do belong more to statistics, numerical mathematics, or operations research [12]. Although this is true for many applications in inpatient or outpatient care, the influence of the specific medical problem is much stronger than in public health.

2. Informatics

Among the fields mentioned in Section 1.2 overlapping with medical informatics, informatics has a major role. Therefore, a short introduction into its structure and concepts is necessary.

2.1 Structure

Theoretical informatics is that part of informatics related to applied mathematics. The field comprises the structures and possibilities for the description of information and information processing. It consists of the following subfields:

- automata theory
- formal languages
- programming theory.

Practical informatics comprises the general methods of programming computers ("software") and consists of the following subfields:

- operating systems
- programming languages
- compilers
- information systems
- data base systems.

The theoretical foundations of these subfields may also be included in theoretical informatics.

Technical informatics is related to communication engineering and comprises the construction of computers ("hardware").

The above three main subfields of informatics are complemented by **applied informatics** corresponding to numerous applications in science and daily life and denoted according to the "host" science:

- medical informatics
- informatics in economy
- informatics in law
- ...

2.2 Fundamental Concepts

The most important fundamental concepts shall be explained in this section in order to avoid repeated references to the special literature.

2.2.1 Message and Information

A concrete **message** contains abstract **information** [14]. The information is extracted by the application of interpretation rules.

From the message "120" the information "concentration of 120 mg/100 ml" is extracted by the interpretation "number with the unit of measure mg/100 ml". If the attribute "hexoses in serum" is additionally known, then from the message "concentration of 120 mg/100 ml" the information "concentration of 120 mg/100 ml hexoses in serum" is extracted.

The notions of message and information are not clearly defined. The same transmission may be merely a message or it may contain some specific information, depending on external knowledge. Different messages may contain the same information (high blood pressure, hypertension), and the same message may contain different information depending on the interpretation rules (hippocampus: name of a genus or part of the brain).

The notion of information is so strongly embodied in colloquial language that virtually everybody has an idea of its meaning, but it cannot be precisely defined. This can easily be seen when the same statement is called "informative" by one and "not informative" by another. In everyday communication, "information" means learning unknown facts or acquisition of knowledge. In this sense, the statement "pneumonia is an inflammation of the lung" has no information for a physician.

The colloquial notion of information is related to the colloquial notion of probability. If the result of a test is "probable", on the basis of prior knowledge, then it contains less "information" than if it is "improbable". The statement "hyperglycemia" contains less information if the physician already knows of a glycosuria.

In a **communication system** (Fig. 2.1 and Section 6.3.1), a **message source** selects a message from a set of possible messages for transmission to a **message target**. Because transmission is a physical process needing time, a **transmitter** has to convert the message into a temporal variation (**signal**) of a physical quantity (**signal parameter**). The signal reaches the **receiver** via the (transmission) **channel** where it has to be reconverted to reconstruct the message.

During communication of a human speaker (message source) with a human listener (message target) the message is converted by the speech apparatus (transmitter) into acoustic waves (signal). The waves are transmitted through the air (channel) and are reconstructed by the ear (receiver).

A practical communication system is frequently a chain. The message is passed from target to target by **exchangers** using different signals until it reaches the final destination.

The acoustic waves are converted into mechanical vibrations of the tympanic membrane and via additional stations into electric impulses along nerve fibers until the message is finally processed in the brain.

The message converted by the message source and the message reconverted by the message target may not be identical, because **disturbances** may occur at every element of a communication system (Fig. 2.1).

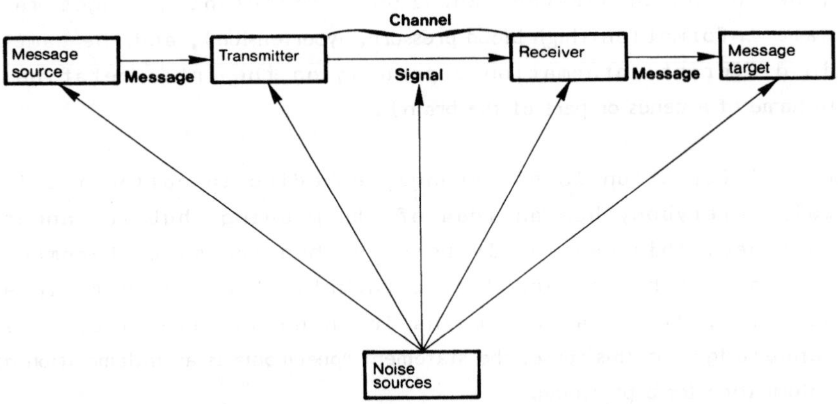

Fig. 2.1: Schema of a communication system

If a cardiac murmur is auscultated, then other noises may be overlaid, the origin of which is also the heart. But there may also be disturbances in the channel due to contamination by, for example, respiratory or intestinal sounds, or by sounds generated outside the body. Disturbances at the receiver may result from an affection of hearing. Finally, the transformation of the signal received may be disturbed, because the examiner does not know exactly how to concentrate his attention on the murmur, and consequently does not "hear" it.

The **semantic** level of information transmission corresponds to the above-mentioned **technical** or **syntactic** level of message transmission. The message source assigns a meaning to the message. Even if the message exchange is free of disturbances, then the information exchange is free of errors only if the message target reads the same meaning out of the message.

In other words, the message source and the message target have to agree on the interpretation rules.

The ability to recognize cardiac murmurs by auscultation can be learned by experience. This does not guarantee that a murmur is correctly interpreted (e.g., interpretation "defect of aortic valve"). Education in medicine is primarily directed towards teaching correct interpretations.

Syntactic and semantic levels of information are complemented by a **pragmatic** level. The transmission of a message is intended to induce a certain reaction in the message target. Whether this reaction is achieved depends on other factors going far beyond the correct interpretation of a message.

Upon examining a patient who is transferred to the hospital for an appendectomy, a surgeon will certainly interpret the message "acute appendicitis" correctly. But, whether this message triggers the desired operation depends on many other factors.

Like other mathematical models, an exact definition of "information" does not consider every aspect of the real situation. But the definition given in the following sections depends heavily on the concept of "known"; its degree of abstraction should not discourage the physician whose work consists mostly of the acquisition of information and the decisions based thereon.

2.2.1.1 Events, Probability

In colloquial language, probability is a measure of the incidence of events. Thus, the event "drop in blood pressure" in a patient with hypertension is "probable" if he is administered a diuretic drug. These intuitive probabilities are learned from experience, as the relative frequencies, with which the respective events were realized in comparable situations in the past.

A test may have the possible results $e_1, e_2, \ldots$. Their totality makes up the **set S of possible results**. Every (sub)set of possible results is an **event**.

The ESR-test may have the possible results $e_1 = 0, e_2 = 1, e_3 = 2, \ldots$. An event may be the union of e_8 to e_{12} (event " normal ESR").

If a test results in an element of an event A, then the event A "occurs".

The **probability** of an event A is a real number assigned to A and denoted by P(A). Probabilities have to obey the following three axioms of

KOLMOGOROV, which correspond to characteristics of relative frequencies:

(1) $P(A) \geq 0$

(2) $P(S) = 1$

(3) $P(A \cup B) = P(A) + P(B)$ for $A \cap B = \emptyset$.

These axioms can easily be illustrated by the distribution of masses (Fig. 2.2). Mass points correspond to the possible results and the quantity of a mass corresponds to the probability. Axiom (1) means that quantities are non-negative real numbers, axiom (2) is a normalization such that the total quantity is equal to 1, and axiom (3) means that the total quantity in two non-overlapping parts is equal to the sum of the individual quantities.

From these axioms follows for two arbitrary events, A and B (Fig. 2.2):

$$P(A \cup B) = P(A) + P(B) - P(A \cap B).$$

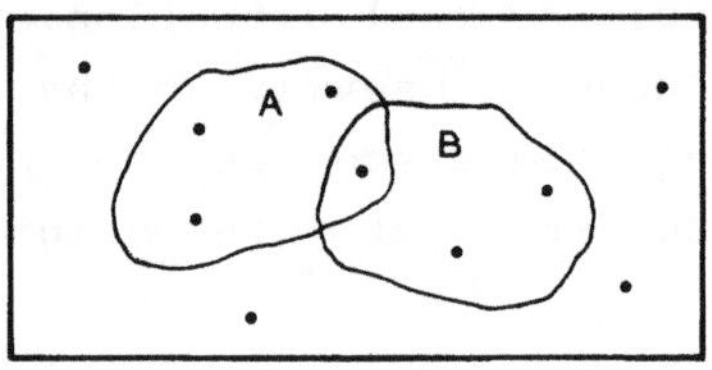

Fig. 2.2: Model with 10 possible results and the events A and B. If every possible event has equal probability, then P(A)=0.4 and P(B)=0.3

These definitions hold for arbitrary probability distributions, but the most interesting cases here are finite sets of possible results. A specialization of this class is that the same probability is assigned to every possible result. This theory has been introduced by LAPLACE. It is especially easy to illustrate and will, therefore, be used to introduce the most important notions. The reader is referred to [85] and Chapter 10 for explanation of the set-theoretic concepts.

Because a possible result is itself an event (**elementary event**), in a model with equal probabilities the probability of an event is computed by simple counting. In this special case it follows from axioms (2) and (3):

$$1 = P(S) = P\left(\bigcup_{i=1}^{n} e_i\right) = \sum_{i=1}^{n} P(e_i) = n \cdot P(e_i) \quad (i=1,2,\ldots,n),$$

and, therefore,

$$P(e_1) = P(e_2) = \ldots = P(e_n) = \frac{1}{n} .$$

If there are k possible results in an event A, then from axiom (3) is $P(A) = \frac{k}{n}$ (number of favorable results divided by the number of possible results).

The abstractly defined probabilities and the empirical relative frequencies are related by the **theorem of large numbers**. This theorem states that the relative frequency of an event converges under certain conditions to the probability of that event as the number of repetitions approaches infinity. The theorem of large numbers also justifies the use of relative frequencies calculated in tests as estimators for the generally unknown probabilities [85].

The notion of conditional probability is of particular importance for understanding information processing. B may be an event with $P(B) > 0$. Then the **conditional probability** $P(A|B)$ of an event A given B is the quotient of the probability, with which both A and B occur and the probability, with which B occurs:

$$(2.1) \qquad P(A|B) = \frac{P(A \cap B)}{P(B)} \quad .$$

The conditional probability is a statement concerning the occurence of the event A when it is already known that B has occured.

Again, the model with equally probable elementary events can serve to illustrate conditional probability. If every possible result in Fig. 2.2 has the same probability and if the event B has occured, then there are only three possible results. Among these results, one result is "favorable". That is:

$$P(A|B) = \frac{P(A \cap B)}{P(B)} = \frac{1/10}{3/10} = \frac{1}{3} \; .$$

Two events A and B are **independent** if $P(A|B)=P(A)$; that is, knowledge about event B does not change the knowledge about event A. If the events A and B are independent, then from (2.1) is:

$$(2.2) \qquad P(A|B) = P(A) \quad \text{and} \quad P(A \cap B) = P(A) \cdot P(B).$$

Conditional probabilities have an important role in medicine. For example, risk factors or side-effects are only understandable by considering conditional probabilities.

If S = 'smoking' is a risk factor for a disease D = 'lung cancer', then

$$P(\text{lung cancer}|\text{smoking}) > P(\text{lung cancer}) \quad \text{or} \quad P(D|S) > P(D) .$$

But if $P(D|S) = P(D)$, then D and S are independent and S is not a risk factor for D.

2.2.1.2 SHANNON's Information Theory

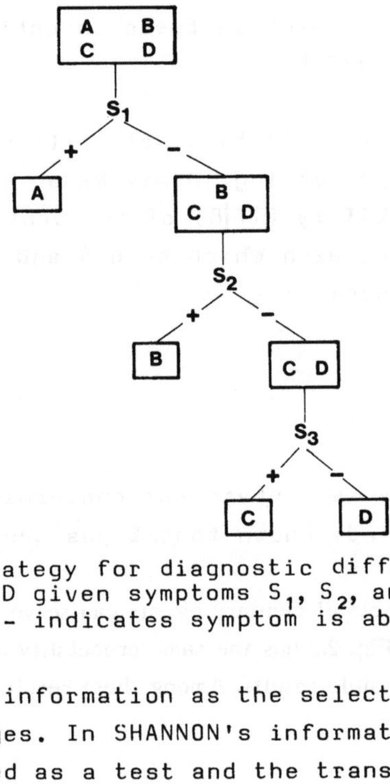

Fig. 2.3: Decision strategy for diagnostic differentiation of the diseases A, B, C, and D given symptoms S_1, S_2, and S_3 (+ indicates symptom is present, - indicates symptom is absent)

Section 2.2.1 defines information as the selection of a message from a set of possible messages. In SHANNON's information theory [72,149] the decision is interpreted as a test and the transmission of a particular message is interpreted as an event, thus emphasizing the **statistical** character of communication processes.

Assume that a patient may have disease A with probability 0.5, disease B with probability 0.25, or diseases C or D each with probability 0.125. The four diseases may be mutually exclusive. Three symptoms S_1, S_2, and S_3 provide diagnostic differentiation, each symptom having two levels (symptom is present/absent). The constellation shall be such that the patient suffers from disease A if S_1 is present, and from diseases B, C, or D if S_1 is absent. If S_2 is present he suffers from disease A or B; otherwise from C or D. If S_3 is present he suffers from C; otherwise from D. Then the strategy in Fig. 2.3 always results in the correct diagnosis. The strategy makes sense, because fewer decisions are necessary in case of the more probable disease than in case of the rarer diseases.

The **decision content** of a disease is measured in bits by the number of required alternative decisions. If the probabilities are such that every alternative decision divides the set of possible results into two equally probable subsets, then following (2.2) the probability P(A) of event A, reached after k decisions, is:

$$P(A) = \left(\frac{1}{2}\right)^k = 2^{-k}.$$

The number of alternative decisions is k=-ld P(A). Generally, the decision content (**information**) I of an event A, occuring with probability P(A), is defined as:

(2.3) $I = -\text{ld}\, P(A)$ (from $0 \leq P(A) \leq 1$ it follows that I is non-negative).

Now if $\{A_1, A_2, \ldots, A_n\}$ is a complete system of events, then the expectation H of the information (**entropy**) is equal to the sum of the informations of the individual events weighted with the respective probabilities:

(2.4) $$H = -\sum_{i=1}^{n} P(A_i) \cdot \text{ld}\, P(A_i) .$$

The maximum entropy of a message source occurs when all n events A_i have the same probability $p_i = P(A_i)$.

Proof: To determine the maximum of H, the partial derivatives of the function

$$H^* = -\sum_{i=1}^{n} p_i \cdot \text{ld}\, p_i + \lambda \cdot \left(1 - \sum_{i=1}^{n} p_i\right)$$

for the p_i have to be calculated (method of LAGRANGE multipliers). This procedure results in the following system of equations, which gives the same maximum for all p_i (e = base of the natural logarithms):

$$\frac{\delta H^*}{\delta p_i} = -\text{ld}\, p_i - \text{ld}\, e - \lambda = 0 \qquad (i=1,2,\ldots,n) .$$

If the probabilities p_i are all equal to $\frac{1}{n}$, then the entropy is

$$(2.5)\qquad \tilde{H} = -\sum_{i=1}^{n} \frac{1}{n}\cdot \mathrm{ld}\,\frac{1}{n} = n\cdot\left(-\frac{1}{n}\cdot \mathrm{ld}\,\frac{1}{n}\right) = \mathrm{ld}\,n\ .$$

The definition (2.3) of "information" is the consequence of the following requirements:

(1) The information I_i with respect to the occurence of an event A_i depends only on the probability $p_i = P(A_i)$:

$$I_i = f(p_i).$$

(2) If two events A_i and A_j are independent, then the information I_{ij} with respect to the occurence both of A_i and A_j is the sum of the informations I_i and I_j. Therefore, it follows from (2.2):

$$I_{ij} = f(p_i\cdot p_j) = f(p_i) + f(p_j).$$

This functional equation has the solution $f(p) = \log p$. The choice of base 2 for the logarithm determines only a constant factor.

Using the probabilities in the example of Fig. 2.3, the entropy is:

$$H = 0.5\cdot 1 + 0.25\cdot 2 + 0.125\cdot 3 + 0.125\cdot 3 = 1.75\ .$$

If the strategy in Fig. 2.4 instead of Fig. 2.3 is chosen, then the decision content (expectation of the number of alternative decisions) is:

$$L = 0.5\cdot 2 + 0.25\cdot 2 + 0.125\cdot 2 + 0.125\cdot 2 = 2\ .$$

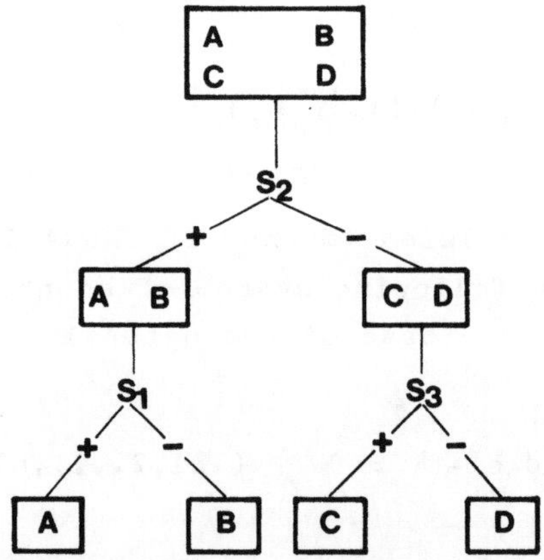

Fig. 2.4: Alternative strategy to the strategy in Fig. 2.3

It can be proved that the decision content L of any strategy satisfies the inequality $L \geq H$ (Section 3.5.1). Therefore, the entropy is the expectation of the optimal strategy. The difference L-H is the **redundancy**.

In the above example, the redundancy is generated by the fact that in Fig. 2.4 an almost useless decision has to be made to reach the frequent event A. This expense cannot be compensated by saving a decision for the rare events C and D.

According to the definitions, the entropy is a measure of the freedom of choice, or, equivalently, the uncertainty about the next occuring event. It increases with the degree of indetermination, i.e., the tendency towards equality of probabilities, and with the number of possible decisions (see (2.5)).

SHANNON's information theory introduces the concept of a message source producing a sequence of characters selected from a set of characters. Event A_i is the selection of the i-th character. The information of a character is greater, the lesser the probability of its selection. Its information is equal to 0 when it is always selected (certain event). The knowledge of the probabilities (or reliable estimates) can be utilized for reduction of the decision costs.

Assume a message source selecting characters from the alphabet of 26 letters. The sequence may be abcdabcdabcdabcd ...

If we assume that every character is selected with equal probability 1/26, then the decision content L is from (2.5)

$$L = \mathrm{ld}\ 26 \simeq 4.7 .$$

But, if we recognize that only the four characters a to d occur and with equal probability, then a strategy can be developed with the decision content

$$L = \mathrm{ld}\ 4 = 2 .$$

If the regularity of the sequence is utilized, then the costs can be further decreased. For example, the integration of the group abcd into the event A results in a message source always producing the certain event A.

This results from the dependence among the possible results a, b, c, and d. If we know one character in the above sequence, then we know, which character can follow, and which character cannot. If the last character sent is a, then for the next character follows from (2.1)

$P(a|a) = P(c|a) = P(d|a) = 0$ and $P(b|a) = 1$.

Thus, redundancy in a decision strategy is generated by interrelated events. The stronger the dependence the more clearly a **cluster** or an **order** is exhibited. An extreme case is an event with a conditional probability of 1.

Fig. 2.5 contains two distributions of 16 points each. The distribution on the left side can be more easily recognized and remembered, because it is quickly assigned to a class (squares). The position of every point is determined by the determination of a point, a direction, and the number of points in a direction.

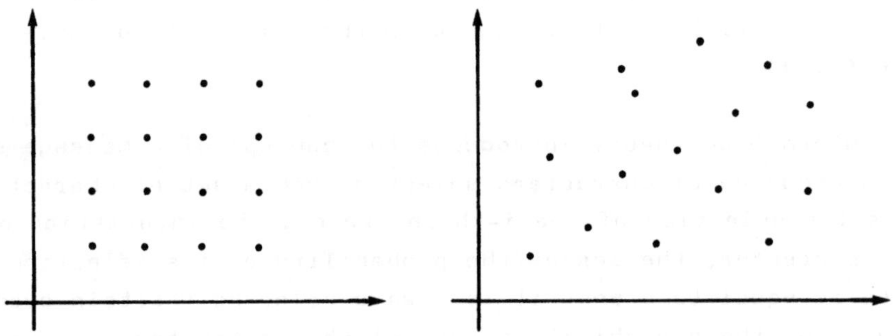

Fig. 2.5: Regular (left) and irregular (right) distribution of points

From every-day experience we know that recognition and utilization of redundancy saves work. Even children employ this experience to learn as economically as possible. Furthermore, consideration of redundancy helps in the understanding of many scientific principles.

The desire for systematization and classification is directly derivable from this experience. Classification produces clusters and makes the recognition and utilization of redundancy possible. If different events can be integrated into the same class, then all we need to remember is the class membership. Hierarchic classification utilizes the fact that in a complex system of attributes the differences between classes are easier to remember than the detailed definitions. This approach governs many different areas such as medical diagnosis (Section 3.5), development of "high level" programming languages (Section 2.2.6.1), systems analysis, or maintenance of medical records (Section 5.1.3.1).

The organization of medical records is especially well-suited to illustrate the problems related to this economy. If we start to create a complete medical record, we find that the number of medical attributes is infinite. Therefore, we restrict the medical record to an enumeration of the differences between the patient and a "normal" state. Everybody knows (or assumes) that the patient has a head, trunk, and extremities, facts which need not be mentioned explicitly, because they would contain no information. But at this point pragmatics has to be considered. The physician entering messages into the medical record has a subjective idea of what he thinks is self-evident. This idea is not necessarily identical with the idea of a colleague or even his own idea at a later time. In other words, the information available when entering data is different from the information when retrieving the same data.

Another aspect of redundancy affects planning, operation, and frequently failure of computer-supported problem solutions. Recognition and utilization of redundancy is an intellectual achievement possibly requiring a considerable amount of knowledge, about which only very few facts are known. Therefore, satisfactory replacement of human achievements in this area requires explicit storage of knowledge, for which appropriate methods are missing to a large extent, or they require a considerable increase in the data base, frequently causing the failure of such projects (Section 5.1.2.3).

Redundancy may also be utilized for the recognition and correction of errors (Section 5.2.2).

Natural language has a considerable redundancy. It makes possible the "understandnig fo distorted texts and the error corerciton".

2.2.2 Languages

Human communication is normally based on a **language.** A language consists of elements (graphemes in a written language, phonemes in a spoken language) arranged using certain rules in syllables, words, phrases, or sentences. The elements of a language are **characters** from a **character set**. A character set is an **alphabet** when an order of the characters is defined.

In most written languages a character is a letter (but note, for example, the Chinese symbolic characters). In the genetic code a character set is realized, which differs from written languages. It consists of the characters "adenine", "cytosine", "guanine", and "thymine". This set is not an alphabet, because no order is defined.

Character sets consisting of exactly two characters are especially important in informatics ("binary" character set). A character is a **binary digit** (**bit**). For example, binary character sets are the pairs "yes/no", "true/false", or "0/1".

Morphology, as defined in linguistics, comprises the rules for word construction from characters. **Syntax** comprises the rules for the construction of larger language units, such as phrases or sentences, from smaller units (words, phrases). **Semantics** is concerned with the meaning expressed by elements of the language. While these three subfields are mainly independent of the individuals engaged in the communication process, **pragmatics** includes speaker and listener considering the common knowledge of the two individuals involved.

A **symbol** is a character combined with its meaning. We may use the symbols A, C, G, and T to "symbolize" the 4 nucleotide bases of the genetic character set.

A **word** is a character sequence interpreted as a unit in a certain context [DIN 44300], or the "smallest self-contained carrier of meaning" [48]. These definitions allow every word to be interpreted as a character on a higher level. Then the character set is made up of the total word set of the language.

Coding is a set of rules for mapping messages from one character set to messages from another character set.

A coding for the attribute "sex" with the levels "male" and "female" are the mapping rules

"male" ⟶ ♂, "female" ⟶ ♀.

Practical reasons for the coding of messages may be:

- secrecy, i.e., reduction of the set of people able to correctly interpret a message,
- compression of messages, i.e., reduction of redundancy (third to fifth lumbar vertebra → L3-L5),
- mapping of semantic relations into formally representable and easier processable relations (Section 3.4.4).

2.2.3 Discretization

A **digital** message consists of single characters. Examples of non-digital or **analog** messages are curves or images. Frequently, it is necessary to map these messages into digital messages for processing (**analog-digital-conversion**). This is done by scanning and quantization.

Combination of scanning and subsequent quantization results in the representation of a non-digital message as a character sequence and thus as a digital message (**digitization**).

An essential characteristic of a discretization method is that it can be formally described. Then agreements about parameters (interval length in 1-dimensional scanning, quantum step in quantization) ensure the independence of the resulting digital message of the applier of these methods.

In medicine, discretization is frequently necessary although there are no operational methods available. Many qualitative findings are of this kind, like classification of a palpable enlargement of the liver into different degrees, or staging of malignant tumors.

2.2.3.1 Scanning

A real-valued continuous function of one variable is a simple case of a non-digital message (Fig. 2.6). The function is scanned by dividing the total interval into subintervals and replacing the function in each subinterval by a constant. This results in a step function. The choice of the constant may depend on the problem (function value in the middle of the subinterval or at one of the boundaries, or mean of the function values). Smaller subintervals preserve the characteristics of the function better. Thus scanning maps a continuous function into a sequence of constants (see classification of data of a continuous attribute [85]).

Images are 2-dimensional non-digital messages. For example, black-and-white images can be interpreted as real-valued functions (light intensity) of two variables (coordinates in the image plane). Such a function can be scanned rectangularly (Fig. 2.7) (see contingency-tables for the data of two classified continuous attributes [85]).

2.2.3.2 Quantization

For quantization, the set of real numbers is decomposed into intervals of equal size t (**quantum step**), and every number r is replaced by the multiple of t located in the same interval as r.

For example, quantization is performed when enzyme activities are measured in international units. An international unit corresponds to a quantum step.

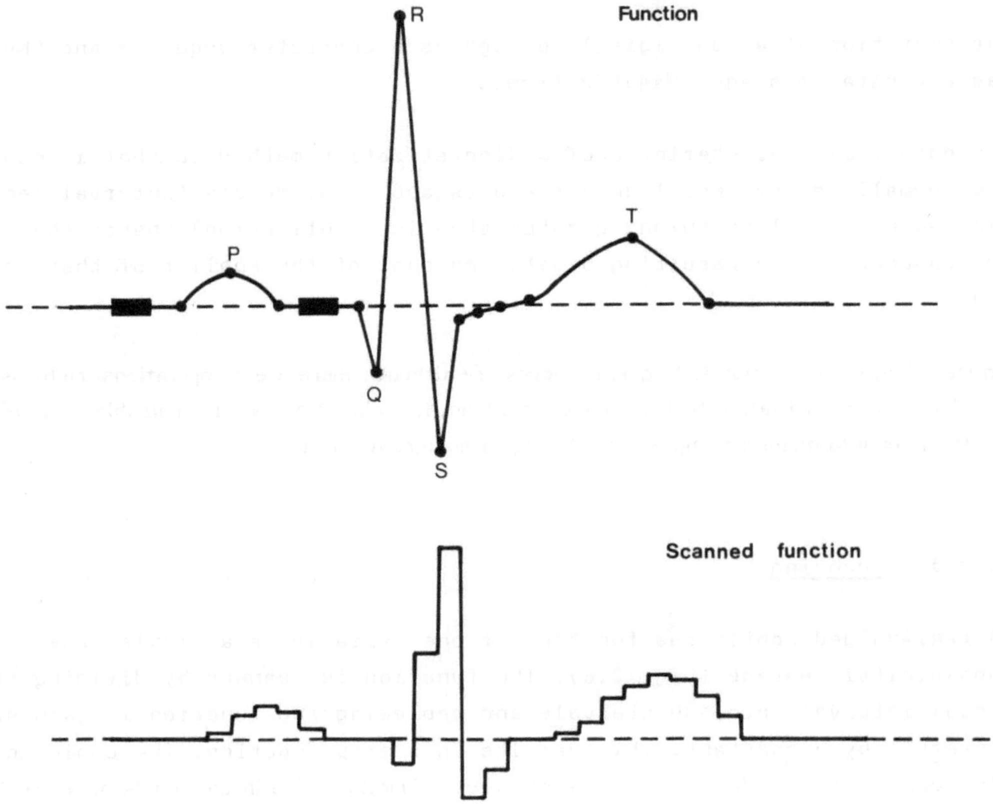

Fig. 2.6: ECG-scanning

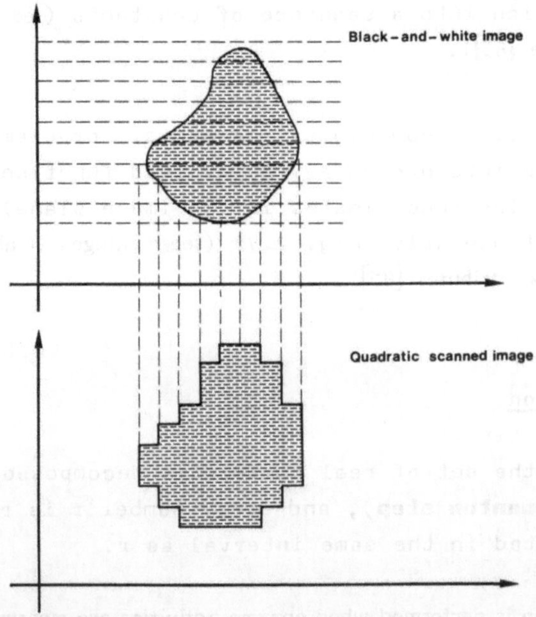

Fig. 2.7: Quadratic scanning

2.2.4 Message Processing and Information Processing

The following considerations are restricted to digital messages. Because each digital message can be interpreted as a single character, a rule ν for mapping a message N_i from a message set $\mathbb{N}$ onto a message N'_i from a message set $\mathbb{N}'$ can be interpreted as coding.

There may be interpretation rules α and α' for mapping the message set $\mathbb{N}$ into the information set $\mathbb{I}$ and the message set $\mathbb{N}'$ into the information set $\mathbb{I}'$. Therefore, each message $N_i \in \mathbb{N}$ corresponds to an information $I_i = \alpha(N_i) \in \mathbb{I}$ as well as to an information $I'_i = \alpha'(\nu(N_i)) \in \mathbb{I}'$:

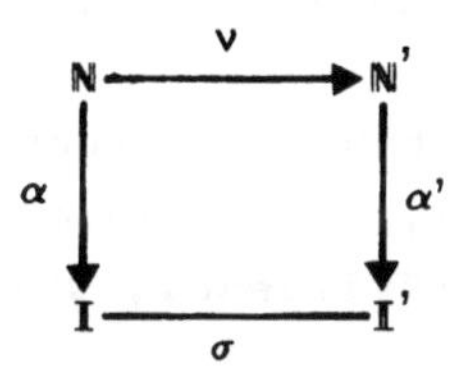

If the mapping α is irreversible, then there are messages $N_i \neq N_j$ and $\alpha(N_i) = \alpha(N_j)$. If $\alpha'(\nu(N_i)) = I'_i \neq I'_j = \alpha'(\nu(N_j))$, then the relation σ between $\mathbb{I}$ and $\mathbb{I}'$ is not a mapping.

If σ is a mapping, then the rule ν is **information preserving** and σ is a rule for **information processing**. A **reversible coding** is distinguished from a **selection** by the fact that σ is reversible. A reversible coding is a **compression** when the size of $\mathbb{N}'$ is smaller than the size of $\mathbb{N}$ (Table 2.1).

Coding	$\mathbb{N}$	$\xrightarrow{\nu}$	$\mathbb{N}'$
Reversible coding	kidney pelvis pelvis renalis	→ →	pelvis renalis kidney pelvis
Selection	kidney medulla kidney cortex	→ →	kidney kidney
Compression	kidney cortex cortex renalis	→ →	cortex renalis cortex renalis

Table 2.1: Examples of different codings

2.2.5 Algorithms

For message processing, $\mathbf{N} \xrightarrow{v} \mathbf{N}'$, the rule v has to be defined such that the transition of a message N_i into a message N'_i requires a finite number of steps. For each step the succeeding step has to be defined (flow diagram). An **algorithm** is a description of the conditions and of the order for transforming a message N_i into a message N'_i in a finite number of steps.

The simplest case of an algorithm is the listing of every relation $N_i \xrightarrow{v} N'_i$ (i=1,2,...,n). It is theoretically always possible, when the size of **N** is finite. Then the algorithm consists of a single step, namely the replacement of N_i by N'_i. In practical situations, however, the size of **N** is so large that this method is unrealistic.

Because the execution of an algorithm is a process needing time, it may be considered how to find a rule v, which minimizes time. These considerations result in the concept of **efficiency**, which is ignored in a pure mathematical treatment of mappings.

2.2.6 Formal Languages

The theory of formal languages [139] is an essential part of informatics and has many connections with linguistics. The most important concepts and connections are presented here to facilitate comprehension of the formulation of problems and solutions in medical linguistics (Chapter 4).

A **formal language** consists of a set V_T of language characters (**terminal characters**), a set V_N of **syntactic variables** (**non-terminal characters**), a **starting symbol** $Z \in V_N$, and a transitive relation $\Longrightarrow$. The **vocabulary** V is the union of V_T and V_N. V^* may be the set of words composed of characters from V including the null word ϵ. The transitive relation $\Longrightarrow$ is a mapping of V^* into itself such that from

$$a \Longrightarrow b,\ b \Longrightarrow c \text{ it follows } a \Longrightarrow c, \quad a,b,c \in V^* .$$

If $a \Longrightarrow b$, then "b is a **derivative** of a".

The **kernel** of the formal language is the set of words derivable from Z by $\Longrightarrow$. The **syntax** (derivation structure) is the set of all derivations $a \Longrightarrow b$.

The relation $\Longrightarrow$ is the **transitive envelope** of a relation $\longrightarrow$, when the derivation $a \Longrightarrow b$ is generated by a finite sequence:

$$a \longrightarrow b_1 \longrightarrow b_2 \longrightarrow \ldots \longrightarrow b_n = b \ .$$

A pair (a,b) with $a \longrightarrow b$ is a **production.** The element b is said to be "directly derivable" from a. A production is elementary in the sense that it cannot be generated by a sequence of other productions.

A **formal grammar** $\Gamma = (V_T, V_N, Z, P)$ describes a formal language, the syntax of which is used to find all words of the kernel that consist only of terminal symbols. P denotes the set of productions.

The **Semi-THUE** languages form an important special case. In these languages, $xay \longrightarrow xby$ is always derivable from $a \longrightarrow b$, when $(a,b,x,y) \varepsilon V^*$. That is, the character string a can be always replaced by the character string b, independent of the adjacent characters. In other words, $a' \longrightarrow b'$ with $a' = xay$ and $b' = xby$ is a production if and only if b is not derivable from a.

A **context-free grammar** consists only of productions $a \longrightarrow b$ with $a \varepsilon V_N$, $b \varepsilon V^*, b \neq \epsilon$.

Productions with the same left side are frequently put together:

$$\left.\begin{matrix} a \longrightarrow b \\ a \longrightarrow c \end{matrix}\right\} \text{is written as} \quad a \longrightarrow b \,|\, c \quad (b \text{ "or" } c) \ .$$

Because the set of productions can be interpreted as a set of messages with a fixed structure, a grammar can be formulated to describe their structure (grammar of a grammar).

Only one example is presented here. For additional examples see Chapter 4.

$V_N = \{ Z, AP, Adj, P, N \}$, $V_T = \{$ acute, chronic, subacute, inflammation, and $\}$

The set of productions is:

1) $Z \longrightarrow AP$

2) $AP \longrightarrow Adj\ AP \,|\, P\ AP \,|\, N$

3) $Adj \longrightarrow$ acute | chronic | subacute

4) $P \longrightarrow$ and

5) $N \longrightarrow$ inflammation.

Elements of the vocabulary of this language are (the numbers refer to the productions):

$$Z \xrightarrow{1} AP \xrightarrow{2} N \xrightarrow{5} \text{inflammation}$$

$$Z \xrightarrow{1} AP \xrightarrow{2} Adj\ \ AP \xrightarrow{3} \text{acute}\ \ AP \xrightarrow{2} \text{acute}\ \ N \xrightarrow{5} \text{acute inflammation}$$

$$Z \xrightarrow{1} AP \xrightarrow{2} Adj\ \ AP \xrightarrow{2} Adj\ \ P\ \ AP \xrightarrow{3,4,2,3} \text{acute and subacute}\ \ AP \xrightarrow{2} \ldots\ .$$

In addition, elements can be created, which make "no sense", like

$$Z \xrightarrow{1} AP \xrightarrow{2} Adj\ \ AP \xrightarrow{3} \text{acute}\ \ AP \xrightarrow{2} \text{acute}\ \ P\ \ AP \xrightarrow{4,2,5} \text{acute and inflammation.}$$

In the example, the **deductive** direction from the starting symbol to the elements of the language is used. The reverse direction (**verifying** direction) from the utterance back to the starting symbol Z permits the decision, whether or not an utterance is an element of the language. By indicating the way back to Z it is at the same time an analysis of the element.

2.2.6.1 Programming Languages

Programming languages are used to formalize algorithms such that, on the one hand, they approach the human kind of arguing and thinking and, on the other hand, they are processable by computer systems.

In programming languages, a message N together with the related information I, $N \xrightarrow{\alpha} I$, is an **object**. N is the **denotation** and I is the **value** of the object (Section 5.1).

The denotation "38.5" has the value "thirty eight point five". If this is a real number, then the denotation "3.85 · 10" has the same value.

Operations in programming languages are the rules of an algorithm for the transformation of messages.

As defined in the preceding sections, an algorithm is essentially an organized prescription for the transformation of characters. For example, mathematical operations, like "addition of two integers", can be broken down into a sequence of elementary operations for replacement of characters. E.g., if the operation "addition of two integers" and the respective algorithm are put down in writing, then one can interpret both forms as messages and the transition from the message "a + b" to the written form of the algorithm as message processing. This interpretation makes possible a comfortable notation for standard operations, like "a + b", instead of the often obscure form of the elementary character transition. In order to do this, an algorithm has to be formulated just once, mapping the notation "a + b" into the level of character transition. One level higher, multiplication of two integers may be represented by an algorithm utilizing the addition of integers as the elementary operation.

Thus, on different levels operations of increasing complexity may be defined, for which the operations on lower levels serve as elementary operations.

This is the principle of programming languages. Their elements depend mainly on the available elementary operations and on the spectrum of algorithms to be formulated as easily as possible.

Such "high level" programming languages include:

ALGOL	(ALGOrithmic Language) [159,165]
ALPHA	(data manipulation language) [30]
BASIC	(Beginner's All-purpose Symbolic Instruction Code) [146]
COBOL	(COmmon Business Oriented Language) [2, DIN 66028]
FORTRAN	(FORmula TRANslation) [3,49,50, DIN 66027]
LISP	(LISt Processing language) [104]
PL/I	(Programming Language/I) [68,176]
SEQUEL	(a Structured English QUEry Language) [11,25].

The formulation of an algorithm in such a language is called a **program**. Its elements are the **instructions**. Special message processing programs (**compiler**) translate the program into a sequence of elementary operations, which can be understood and processed by a computer system.

2.2.7 Architecture of Digital Computers

Computers are machines for automatic processing of messages. Digital computers and analog computers are distinguished by the kind of messages they process. The following discussion is limited to digital computers because of their practical significance.

The abstract level, on which computers are discussed in automata theory [78], is not suitable here, because a physician who is interested in medical informatics should primarily be informed about the most important concepts in a similar fashion to using a modern desk-top calculator.

Data are "read in" via **input units**. They are processed in the **central processing unit** (CPU) and the results are "written" onto **output units** (Fig. 2.8).

Input units include card reader, paper tape reader, magnetic tape unit, magnetic disk unit, mark sense form reader, document reader, and display unit with light pen and/or keyboard. Output units include high speed printer, card punch, paper tape punch, magnetic tape unit, magnetic disk unit, and display.

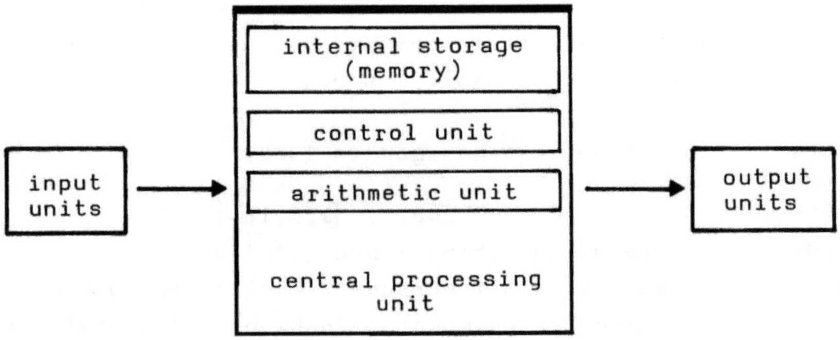

Fig. 2.8: Components of a computer

The CPU consists of the **control unit**, the **arithmetic unit**, and the **internal storage**. In the internal storage not only data but also instructions are stored. The control unit controls the processing of data and instructions in the arithmetic unit, which processes the instructions. The control unit also ensures that the data used as operands are "fetched" from the internal storage and made available to the arithmetic unit. Finally, the results are stored in appropriate locations in the internal storage.

Arithmetic operations include addition, subtraction, multiplication, and division of numbers. **Logical** operations govern the comparison of numbers (greater than, equal to, less than) or character strings (equal to, not equal to).

The **internal** storage is complemented by various **external** storage media, like punch card, paper tape, magnetic tape, and magnetic disk. They differ with respect to capacity, reusability, access time (time needed to move data into or out of storage), costs, and in the possible access modes (**sequential**, as on magnetic tapes or **direct**, as on magnetic disks).

2.2.8 Operating Modes of Digital Computers

A computer may be operated in various **modes**, which can be combined.

In **batch**-mode, the user cannot change the sequence of steps during execution of his program. The program is submitted to the computer on a computer-readable data medium, e.g., punch cards or paper tape. The computer executes the programs of different users concurrently and independently of each other. The order of execution depends on the availability of resources (main storage, input units, output units). In a simple system the order is sequential, e.g., first-in-first-out. In a more complex system the program of a user can be executed while at the same time data are read in for another program from an input unit. The user has no direct control on the execution order of programs submitted to the system.

In **time-sharing**-mode, the user accesses a computer via a **terminal**, similar to an electric typewriter or a TV-monitor with a keyboard. Many terminals may simultaneously be connected to a computer. The user carries out a "dialog" with the computer system and influences the execution of his program via input of data, which may depend on the execution state. This mode is more convenient for the user than batch-mode, saves time in many applications, and makes **man-machine interaction** possible. In this mode, the computer is assigned the more formal (syntactic) tasks and the human is assigned the more semantic tasks. Because a user usually needs more time to accomplish his tasks when compared with the processing speed of a computer, it is appropriate that several programs are executed alternately (i.e., multiplexed) instead of sequentially. The internal processing speed is so fast that virtually each user is served simultaneously and conveys the appearance that he has complete control of the systems resources.

In **process**-mode (**real time**-mode), automatic instruments are connected to the computer (such as analyzers in the laboratory, instruments in nuclear medicine). A particular characteristic of such "process-computers" is the automatic interruption of execution triggered by signals on signal interface lines. In general, signal acquisition has priority over other processing, because data must not be lost and instruments usually cannot store these data. Data processing programs can be started depending on the input signals and can themselves generate signals for the control of instruments. Thus, a closed cycle of function and control can be built.

2.2.9 Computer-Supported Problem Solving

Several fundamental remarks concerning the use of computers are presented in this section. It is necessary to clearly formulate the problem and the desired solution. This statement is in its general form almost trivial. Nevertheless, in practical situations it may be very difficult to achieve.

Developing a computer-supported solution to a problem may be divided into several phases (Fig. 2.9). Problem definition is based on an exact description of the information required as the result of processing. Ultimately, this description specifies the types of data to be acquired. The connecting link between data input and information retrieval is a program, in which the algorithms are formulated.

Systems analysis defines the interface requirements of a program (input data, input time, output data, output time, mode of data presentation, ...). It leads from the analysis of the actual situation to a plan of organization of the problem solution, which includes the **algorithms** in its most detailed version [174].

Formulation of the algorithms in the chosen programming language is the actual **programming**. This phase is followed by a **program test** and an error correction phase (i.e., debugging). Modern systems and programming techniques provide formal error checks concurrently with programming [43]. Program test is followed by the **implementation**.

Such a linear sequence of the different phases is rare. In complicated cases, particularly if tasks are to be partitioned between human individuals and computer, the use of computers frequently leads to alterations in the users behavior. This may go so far that shifts in the partition of tasks are required, which enforce a repetition of systems analysis.

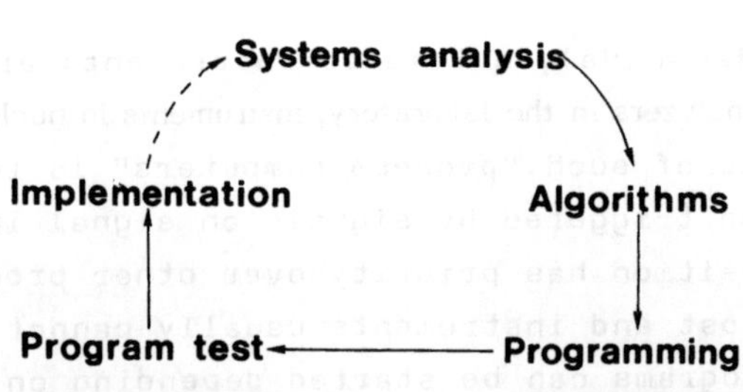

Fig. 2.9: Interrelations between phases during computer-supported problem solving

3. Classification

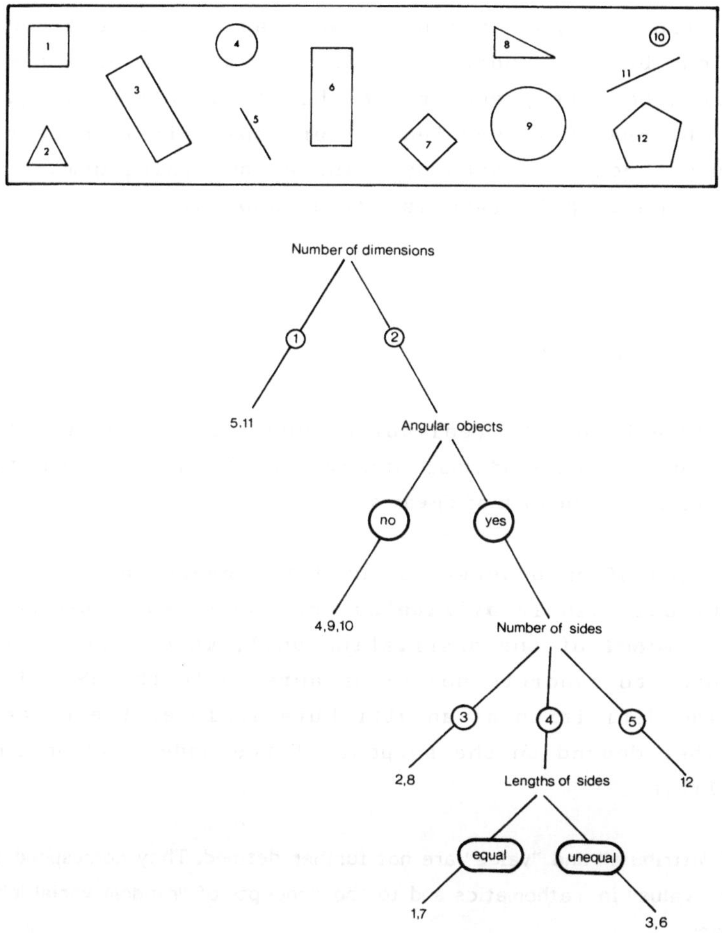

Fig. 3.1: Classification of a set of real world objects

The notion of classification comprises very different applications, but they all can be reduced to a common basic form:

- A set of objects of the real world is given. They are classified into subsets such that elements in the same subset have in common as much or as specific attributes as possible and elements in different subsets differ as much as possible (Fig. 3.1).

The attributes for the classification of the objects in Fig. 3.1 are presented at the branches of the schema. The individual denotations (i.e., numbers) of the objects are presented at the end of the respective chains. If the subsets are respectively denoted, then the real world contains: 2 line segments, 3 circles, 2 triangles, 2 squares, 2 rectangles, and 1 pentagon.

The objective of classification is an **order** by recognition of common features of objects and by recognition of clusters. As explained in Section 2.2.1.2, this objective is so fundamental in information processing that the broad spectrum of applications as well as of sciences contributing to the solutions becomes understandable. The most important methods for medical applications are presented in this chapter without going into great depth. The reader interested in more specific literature is referred to the methods of: taxonomy, cluster analysis, game theory, decision theory, and computer(-assisted) diagnosis.

3.1 Observation Units, Attributes

We designate objects of the real world henceforth as **observation units.** Examples of observation units are individuals (zoologic classifications), atoms (natural system of elements), or concepts (classification of diseases).

For the modelling of an observation unit not every possible aspect is interesting, but only single **attributes** and their **relations** to each other. These create a **model** of the observation unit, which can be used as long as its responses to concrete questions agree with the experience in the real world. The definition of an attribute includes the enumeration of the **values.** They depend on the purpose of the model and on the observation possibilities.

The concepts of "attribute" and "value" are not further defined. They correspond to the concepts of "variable" and "value" in mathematics and to the concepts of "random variable" and "possible result" in statistics.

The set of values of each attribute has to induce a **decomposition** of the set of observation units [85] to make sure that each observation unit is assigned exactly one value.

The attributes are classified into types according to the applicable methods. These types are given various designations in the literature.

The values of **qualitative** attributes are concepts. Qualitative attributes are further classified into **nominal** attributes, when the values are categories, for which no natural ordering exists ("sex" with values "male" and "female") and in **ordinal** attributes, when the values are ordered ("gradation of a disease" with values "mild", "moderate", and "severe").

The values of **quantitative** attributes are numbers a priori, which for a **continuous** attribute are determined by measuring a (theoretically) continuous quantity ("blood pressure" in mm Hg), while values of a **discrete** attribute are obtained by counting ("number of appointments").

The values of non-continuous attributes are called **levels.**

3.1.1 Attribute Structures

In this section a short introduction into a theory is presented, which is based on **lattice theory** [15] and which can be used to describe formally relations between attributes (**deep structure**) [67]. Besides the various applications in the design of clinical trials, such descriptions are particularly important for the formal description of the classification of concepts [111].

An **ordered set**

$$\mathbf{S} = \{x, y, \ldots\}$$

is a set on which an **ordering relation** "$\leq$" ("smaller than") is defined, i.e., a relation with the following characteristics for all $x, y, z \in \mathbf{S}$:

(1) $x \leq x$ (**reflexivity**),
(2) $x \leq y \wedge y \leq x \rightarrow x = y$ (**antisymmetry**),
(3) $x \leq y \wedge y \leq z \rightarrow x \leq z$ (**transitivity**).

An **upper bound** of a subset **T** of **S** is an element $x \in \mathbf{S}$ with

$$t \leq x \quad \text{for all } t \in \mathbf{T}.$$

The **least upper bound** x_ℓ is an upper bound with

$$x_\ell \leq x \quad \text{for all upper bounds } x.$$

The notions of (**greatest**) **lower bound** are defined dually.

A **lattice L** is an ordered set any two of whose elements, x and y, have a greatest lower bound, $x \sqcap y$, and a least upper bound, $x \sqcup y$.

We use here the symbols $\leq$, $\sqcup$, and $\sqcap$, but it must be kept in mind that these symbols do not necessarily indicate "inclusion" or the set operations "union" and "intersection", respectively.

The operations $\sqcup$ and $\sqcap$ have the following characteristics:

$$\left.\begin{array}{l} x \sqcup x = x \\ x \sqcap x = x \end{array}\right\} \quad (\textbf{idempotency}),$$

$$\left.\begin{array}{l} x \sqcup y = y \sqcup x \\ x \sqcap y = y \sqcap x \end{array}\right\} \quad (\textbf{commutativity}),$$

$$\left.\begin{array}{l} (x \sqcup y) \sqcup z = x \sqcup (y \sqcup z) \\ (x \sqcap y) \sqcap z = x \sqcap (y \sqcap z) \end{array}\right\} \quad (\textbf{associativity}),$$

$$\left.\begin{array}{l} x \sqcap (x \sqcup y) = x \\ x \sqcup (x \sqcap y) = x \end{array}\right\} \quad (\textbf{adjunctivity}).$$

The idempotency can be deduced from the other characteristics.

A lattice $\mathbb{L}$ with the operations $\sqcup$ and $\sqcap$ is called **distributive**, when

$$\left.\begin{array}{l} x \sqcup (y \sqcap z) = (x \sqcup y) \sqcap (x \sqcup z) \\ x \sqcap (y \sqcup z) = (x \sqcap y) \sqcup (x \sqcap z) \end{array}\right\} \quad (\textbf{distributivity}).$$

An element z is called **irreducible**, when

$$x \sqcup y = z \longrightarrow x = z \vee y = z.$$

An expression

$$x = x_0 \sqcup x_1 \sqcup \ldots \sqcup x_k$$

is the **shortest representation** of x, when no operand x_i in the expression can be omitted.

A **unique shortest representation** of each element by irreducible elements is possible, if and only if the lattice is distributive.

The smallest and the greatest elements of the lattice $\mathbb{L}$ will be denoted by e_L^0 and e_L^1, respectively.

An element $a \in \mathbb{L}$ is an **atom**, when

$$e_L^0 \leq x \leq a \longrightarrow x = a \vee x = e_L^0 .$$

Let be $\mathbb{L}'$ a subset of $\mathbb{L}$, which is closed with respect to both operations, i.e.,

$$x, y \in \mathbb{L}' \longrightarrow x \sqcup y \in \mathbb{L}' \wedge x \sqcap y \in \mathbb{L}'.$$

Then $\mathbb{L}'$ is a **sublattice** of $\mathbb{L}$ with the same operations and the same ordering relation defined on the Cartesian product $\mathbb{L}' \times \mathbb{L}'$. If $\mathbb{L}$ is distributive, then $\mathbb{L}'$ is distributive.

A subset $\tilde{\mathbb{L}} \subseteq \mathbb{L}$ of a distributive lattice $\mathbb{L}$ is called **base structure**, when

(1) there is a greatest element $e^1_{\tilde{L}}$ and $\tilde{\mathbb{L}}-e^1_{\tilde{L}}$ is either a base structure or the empty set, or

(2) $\tilde{\mathbb{L}}$ can be broken down into subsets $\tilde{\mathbb{L}}_{(1)},\tilde{\mathbb{L}}_{(2)},\ldots,\tilde{\mathbb{L}}_{(k)}$ such that each subset is a base structure with a greatest element $e^1_{\tilde{L}_{(i)}}$ and

$$e^1_{\tilde{L}_{(i)}} \sqcap e^1_{\tilde{L}_{(j)}} = e^0_L \quad (i \neq j).$$

A population $\mathbb{B}$ of observation units, $\mathbb{B}=\{B_1,B_2,\ldots,B_n\}$, and a set of attributes, $\mathbb{X}=\{X,Y,\ldots\}$, is given. Each attribute is defined by a set of values

$$X = \{x_1,x_2,\ldots,x_v\} .$$

The set $\mathbb{B}(X.x_i)$ is the subset of $\mathbb{B}$ that includes all observation units, on which the value x_i of the attribute X is observed. Let be $\mathbb{B}(X)$ the subset of $\mathbb{B}$ that includes all observation units, on which one of the values of X is observed:

$$\mathbb{B}(X) = \bigcup_{i=1}^{v} \mathbb{B}(X.x_i).$$

Two values x_i and x_j are **disjoint**, if

$$\mathbb{B}(X.x_i) \cap \mathbb{B}(X.x_j) = \emptyset .$$

Two attributes X and Y are **disjoint**, if

$$\mathbb{B}(X) \cap \mathbb{B}(Y) = \emptyset .$$

Let $\mathbb{B}$ be the set of concepts of "inflammations" and "neoplasms", X be the attribute "course" with the values "acute", "subacute", "chronic",... , and Y be the attribute "differentiation" with the values "well differentiated", "moderately differentiated", "poorly differentiated", "undifferentiated",... (Table 5.2, 5.3 in Section 5.1.3.7.2). The values of these attributes are disjoint. Furthermore, these attributes are disjoint, because $\mathbb{B}(X)$ is the set of concepts of "inflammations" and $\mathbb{B}(Y)$ is the set of concepts of "neoplasms".

We restrict tne theory here to attributes with disjoint values. An attribute X is **complete**, when $\mathbb{B}(X)=\mathbb{B}$.

Each attribute X defines a **Boolean sublattice** $\mathbb{W}_X(\subseteq, \cup, \cap)$ of the power set $P(\mathbf{B})$ with the ordering relation **inclusion** and the set operations **union** and **intersection** by :

$$\mathbf{B}(X.x_i) \in \mathbb{W}_X \ (i=1,2,\ldots,v),$$

$$A \in \mathbb{W}_X \longrightarrow \bar{A} \in \mathbb{W}_X,$$

$$A,B \in \mathbb{W}_X \longrightarrow A\cup B \in \mathbb{W}_X \wedge A\cap B \in \mathbb{W}_X,$$

$$e^{0}_{v_X} = \emptyset.$$

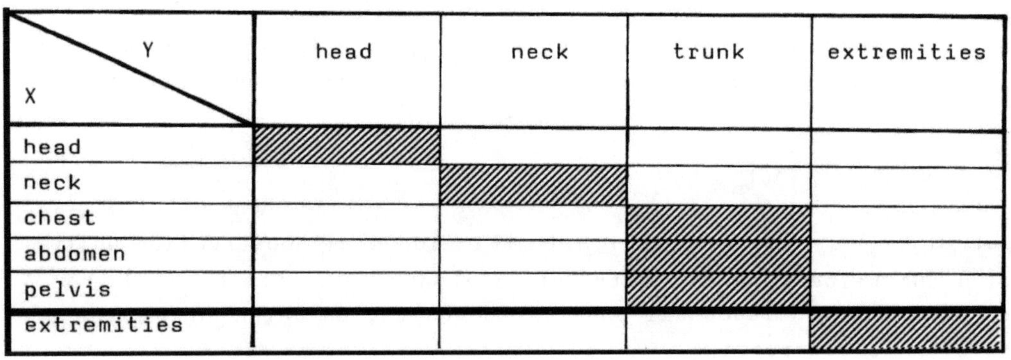

Fig. 3.2: Refinement of the topographic attribute Y by the attribute X. The non-empty intersections are hatched

The **atoms** of $\mathbb{W}_X$ are the sets $\mathbf{B}(X.x_i)$ $(i=1,2,\ldots,v)$.

Attribute values may be attributes themselves (**compound** attributes). An attribute whose values are no attributes is called **primitive** attribute.

For example, the attribute "blood pressure" may have the values "systolic blood pressure" and "diastolic blood pressure". These are attributes whose values are sets of real numbers.

If $x_i = Y$, then

$$\mathbf{B}(X.Y) \subseteq \mathbf{B}(X.x_i)$$

must be accomplished, because the finer values of Y may be observed on less observation units.

A compound attribute (with disjoint values on each level) defines a base structure with $e^0=\emptyset$.

The attribute X is called **refinement** of the attribute Y and, correspondingly, the attribute Y is called **coarsement** of the attribute X, $X \Longrightarrow Y$, when for every value y on any level of Y there is a set of values of X such that

$$\mathbf{B}(X) \subseteq \mathbf{B}(Y) \quad \text{and} \quad \bigcup_i \mathbf{B}(X. \ldots .x_i) = \mathbf{B}(Y. \ldots .y).$$

Let **B** be the set of topographic regions and X and Y be the attributes (Fig. 3.2):

$$X = \{\text{head, neck, chest, abdomen, pelvis, extremities}\},$$
$$Y = \{\text{head, neck, trunk, extremities}\}.$$

Then X is a refinement of Y, $X \Longrightarrow Y$.

Two attributes X and Y are called **equivalent**, when both X is a refinement and a coarsement of Y. Then both attributes define the same lattice.

The relation $\Longrightarrow$ defines on the set $\mathbb{X}$ of attributes or on the set of corresponding Boolean lattices $\mathbb{W}_X$ an order, which can be used to define two operations:

(1) $X * Y$ as the **coarsest refinement**
(2) $X \# Y$ as the **finest coarsement**
} of both attributes.

The set of lattices of P(**B**) is a lattice with respect to the ordering relation $\Longrightarrow$ and these two operations. In general, this lattice is neither distributive nor modular.

In other words:

(1) The relation $\Longrightarrow$ is an ordering relation (i.e., reflexive, antisymmetric, and transitive),
(2) for any two attributes X and Y exists the "least upper bound" $X * Y$, corresponding to $X \sqcup Y$, and the "greatest lower bound" $X \# Y$, corresponding to $X \sqcap Y$.

Two attributes X and Y are (pairwise) **weakly orthogonal**, when $X \# Y$ is an attribute Z with a single value z, i.e., $\mathbf{B}(Z.z)=\mathbf{B}(X) \cup \mathbf{B}(Y)$.

Two attributes X and Y are (pairwise) **orthogonal**, when for all i and j:

$$\mathbf{B}(X.x_i) \cap \mathbf{B}(Y.y_j) \neq \emptyset \quad (i=1,2,\ldots,v_X;\ j=1,2,\ldots,v_Y).$$

For two orthogonal attributes, X and Y, the product $X * Y$ is isomorphic to the Cartesian product $X \times Y$. Pairwise orthogonality induces pairwise weak orthogonality.

Let be X and Y two orthogonal attributes and let X' and Y' be attributes having a subset of the values of X and Y, respectively. Then X' and Y' are also orthogonal.

(Weak) orthogonality of more than two attributes is defined analogously:

> A set $\mathbf{X}=\{X_1,X_2,\ldots,X_s\}$ is (weakly) **orthogonal**, when any two products from disjoint subsets of **X** are pairwise (weakly) orthogonal. Pairwise (weakly) orthogonal attribute sets are not necessarily (weakly) orthogonal.

Let **B** be the set of concepts of "inflammations". Then the attributes "course", "spread", and "circulation alteration", as defined in Table 5.2 (Section 5.1.3.7.2), are orthogonal.

Thus, the product "course" * "spread" corresponds to an attribute with the values:

> {acute and focal, acute and diffuse, acute and multifocal, ...,
> subacute and focal, subacute and diffuse, subacute and multifocal, ...,
> ...}.

The set of attributes observed in an observation unit together with their interrelations forms a model of the observation unit. Usually, one is interested in models, which are possibly simple, i.e., if two models are available, yielding the same information, then the simpler model is preferred. This leads to the problem of selecting an attribute base. Because a unique shortest representation of elements by irreducible elements requires a distributive lattice, one is usually interested in attribute structures, which are distributive with respect to the operations "*" and "#". These lattices are defined by their irreducible elements and the deep structure.

The **deep structure** of an attribute set **X** is defined by the enumeration of

- pairs with X==>Y (i.e., the order of the set of attributes),
- disjoint attributes,
- orthogonal attributes.

An attribute set $\mathbf{X}=\{X_1,X_2,\ldots\}$ is an **attribute base**, when **X** defines a base structure, i.e.:

(1) **X** includes a greatest element e^1_X, i.e., e^1_X is a refinement of each X_j, and $\mathbf{X}-e^1_X$ is an attribute base or the empty set, or

(2) **X** can be broken down into subsets $\mathbf{X}_{(1)},\mathbf{X}_{(2)},\ldots$ such that each subset is an attribute base with a greatest element $e^1_{X_{(i)}}$, and the set $\{e^1_{X_{(1)}},e^1_{X_{(2)}},\ldots\}$ is weakly orthogonal.

An attribute base can be represented as a set of trees (Fig. 3.3):

(1) If $\mathbf{X}$ includes a greatest element, then this element is placed into the single son node. The set $\mathbf{X}-e^1_X$ is treated alike.
(2) If $\mathbf{X}$ can be broken down into subsets, as they are described in the definition, then the node is splitted into a node for each greatest element of the respective subset. The sets $\mathbf{X}_{(i)}-e^1_{X_{(i)}}$ are treated alike.
(3) If there remains only one attribute in a node, then this attribute is broken down into its values. The values must be disjoint. Each value is assigned a node. Values which are attributes are treated alike.

Fractures can be described by the following attributes:

number = $\{1, 2, \ldots\}$,
course = {transverse, oblique, spiral, longitudinal, ...},
surface = {open, closed},
infection = {infected, not infected}.

There are the following relations:

(1) all four attributes have disjoint values,
(2) the set {number, course, surface} is orthogonal,
(3) infection, as it is understood here, is only possible for open fractures.

We can, therefore, find a base structure by defining "surface" as a compound attribute, such that the value "open" is interpreted as an attribute with the values "open infected" and "open not infected" (Fig. 3.3).

But, if the attribute "number" is defined with the values {single, multiple}, then the set is no longer orthogonal. A classification, using this definition of "number" [33], leads to a loss of information for multiple fractures.

The above-explained theory is well-suited for classifying **missing data** (e.g., as to the cause of missing data).

3.1.2 Binary Attributes

Binary (dichotomous) attributes are of special importance in informatics. They are nominal attributes with exactly two levels. Thus, binary attributes describe whether a characteristic is present or absent.

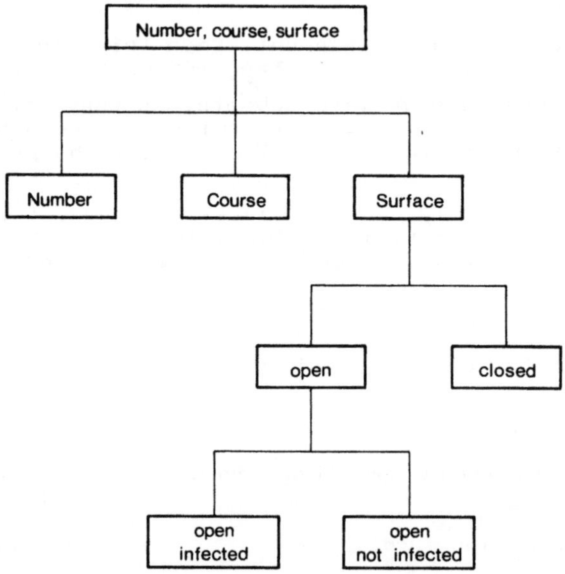

Fig. 3.3: Attribute base for the description of fractures

There are different methods for transforming **non-binary** attributes into binary attributes, which may best be described by **indicator variables** [85]. Transformation into a single binary attribute is, in general, a special **coarsement**.

A qualitative or discrete attribute X may have the levels x_i^*; a continuous attribute X may be classified (Section 2.2.3.1) with the i-th class $(a_{i-1}, a_i]$. Then a random variable Y is defined by:

$$Y = i \quad \text{if } X = x_i^* \quad \text{or} \quad X \in (a_{i-1}, a_i] \; (i=1,2,...,m).$$

An indicator variable M is defined by:

$$M = \begin{Bmatrix} 0, & Y \in I \\ 1, & Y \notin I \end{Bmatrix} \quad , \; I \subseteq \{1,2,...,m\}.$$

A specialization of this method is found in quantitative attributes X:

A quantitative attribute X may be dichotomized by its median. This transformation results in a loss of information. An indicator variable M_D is defined by:

$$M_D = \begin{Bmatrix} 0, & X < \tilde{\mu} \\ 1, & \text{otherwise} \end{Bmatrix} \; .$$

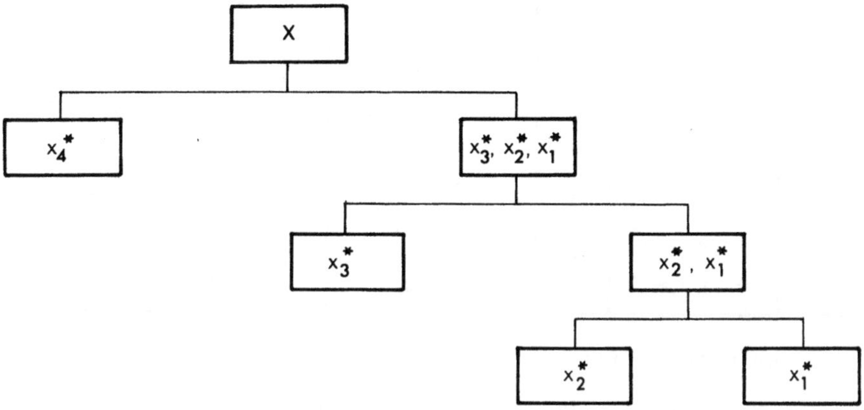

Fig. 3.4: Transformation of an attribute into a compound attribute

In addition, there are some methods, applicable for every attribute type, which replace an attribute X by a set $\{M_1, M_2, \ldots\}$ of indicator variables corresponding to a set of (weakly) orthogonal attributes (Table 3.1):

Method I: m indicator variables are defined by:

$$M_i = \begin{cases} 1, & Y = i \\ 0, & \text{otherwise} \end{cases} \qquad (i=1,2,\ldots,m) \quad .$$

This method leads to a set of attributes with value 1 on disjoint sets of observation units.

Method II: m-1 indicator variables are defined by:

$$M_i = \begin{cases} 1, & Y \leq i \\ 0, & \text{otherwise} \end{cases} \qquad (i=1,2,\ldots,m-1) \quad .$$

This method leads to a set of attributes with value 1 on nested sets of observation units. X is transformed into a compound attribute whose values are sets of the original values of X (Fig. 3.4).

Method III: $\lceil \mathrm{ld}\ m \rceil$ indicator variables are defined by:

$$Y = 1 + \sum_{i=1}^{\lceil \mathrm{ld}\ m \rceil} M_i \cdot 2^{i-1}$$

(representation of Y as a binary number and association of an indicator variable with each position of this number).

This method leads to a set of non-disjoint attributes. This set is weakly orthogonal and is orthogonal, when the number of levels of X is a power of 2.

X		Y	I				II			III	
qualitative/ discrete	continuous		M_1	M_2	M_3	M_4	M_1	M_2	M_3	M_1	M_2
$X = x_1^*$	$X \varepsilon (a_0, a_1]$	1	1	0	0	0	1	1	1	0	0
$X = x_2^*$	$X \varepsilon (a_1, a_2]$	2	0	1	0	0	0	1	1	1	0
$X = x_3^*$	$X \varepsilon (a_2, a_3]$	3	0	0	1	0	0	0	1	0	1
$X = x_4^*$	$X \varepsilon (a_3, a_4]$	4	0	0	0	1	0	0	0	1	1

Table 3.1: Three methods for the replacement of an attribute X by a set of indicator variables. Random variable Y receives the number of the level or the class of X, respectively

3.1.3 Trustworthiness of Data Observation

A **datum** is the value of an attribute observed in a specific observation unit. This concept is frequently confused with the "value" of an attribute: "values" comprise all the possible outcomes, whereas "data" are, in fact, the observed outcomes. For all types of attributes, observation of the data depends on a rule, which makes the assignment of a value possible. Each rule must be explicit in order to obtain data independent of the observer. Frequently, this **operational definition** of data observation cannot be accomplished, as, for example, in such fundamental attributes as "health" with the values "healthy" and "sick".

The **trustworthiness** of data observation is characterized by several measures. If M is a binary attribute with the values E and $\bar{E}$, then the result of data observation in n observation units can be described by a fourfold table (Table 3.2).

	Reality: E	Reality: $\bar{E}$	Sum of rows
Decision E	n_{11}	n_{12}	$n_{1\bullet} = n_{11} + n_{12}$
Decision $\bar{E}$	n_{21}	n_{22}	$n_{2\bullet} = n_{21} + n_{22}$
Sum of columns	$n_{\bullet 1} = n_{11} + n_{21}$	$n_{\bullet 2} = n_{12} + n_{22}$	n

Table 3.2: Result of data observation ("decision") in n observation units for a binary attribute

Important measures for the trustworthiness of data observation are:

$$\textbf{Sensitivity} = \frac{n_{11}}{n_{.1}}$$ (conditional relative frequency of a correct decision given E is present),

$$\textbf{Specifity} = \frac{n_{22}}{n_{.2}}$$ (conditional relative frequency of a correct decision given E is absent).

If data observation is interpreted as a statistical test with the null hypothesis "level E is present", then (1-sensitivity) corresponds to the probability of the error first kind and (1-specifity) corresponds to the probability of the error second kind [85]. In general, both measures are interrelated. Their calculation requires an "outside criterion", which permits the decision whether or not E is present. A measure whose calculation requires no outside criterion is the **reliability** (relative frequency of the **same** decision in independent test repetitions).

Frequently in medicine, **hard** (reliable) data are distinguished from **soft** (unreliable) data. The belief in the greater reliability of quantitative data is based on the feeling that data observation by a machine is in general more reliable than judgement by human. Experience shows that for a good technical device the variability of the data is relatively small in repeated measurements of the same specimen. But the variability of the data caused by the intraindividual variability of the observation unit is considerably greater [97,128]. Therefore, the belief in the reliability of quantitative data is frequently based on a confusion of measured object (worked-up serum) and observation unit (patient).

In principle, the reliability of data is inversely related to the complexity of the corresponding attribute. Examples are compound ordinal attributes mapping a multi-dimensional state into a primitive attribute (Section 5.1).

Describing the "improvement" of a patient with polyarthritis under therapy requires consideration of attributes such as X-ray findings, clinical findings, laboratory tests, and complaints. Even if operational definitions are available for the "subattributes", they will require a general agreement as to their weights, in order to make reliable statements of "improved", "unchanged", or "worse" (Section 3.3.2.2.2).

A **relation** is defined by the **object triplet**: (observation unit, attribute, value). Because object triplets can be nested, i.e., hierarchically related, relations can be utilized to form complex data structures (Section 5.1).

3.1.4 Models

The theory, introduced in Section 3.1.1, can be used to develop construction principles for modelling observation units by attributes (e.g., principles for the classification of concepts).

Given a set $\mathbf{B}$ of observation units, a lattice $(\mathbf{L},\subseteq)$ contained in the power set $P(\mathbf{B})$ with the operators $\cup$ (union) and $\cap$ (intersection), a lattice $(\mathbf{C},\leq)$ with the operators $\sqcup$ and $\sqcap$, and an injection $\mathbf{C} \xrightarrow{\varphi} \mathbf{L}$. The lattice $\mathbf{C}$ with the injection φ is called a **model** $(\mathbf{C},\varphi)$ for $\mathbf{B}$, if:

(1) $\varphi(x) \in \mathbf{L}$ for each $x \in \mathbf{C}$,

(2) for each $\ell \in \mathbf{L}$ there is an $x \in \mathbf{C}$ with $\varphi(x)=\ell$,

(3) for each $x,y \in \mathbf{C}$ is $\varphi(x \sqcup y) = \varphi(x) \cup \varphi(y)$,

(4) for each $x,y \in \mathbf{C}$ is $\varphi(x \sqcap y) = \varphi(x) \cap \varphi(y)$.

In practical situations one is interested in constructing models based on a certain, mostly incomplete body of knowledge concerning $\mathbf{L}$:

> Let $\mathbf{C}^*$ be a set and φ^* a mapping $\mathbf{C}^* \xrightarrow{\varphi^*} \mathbf{L}^*$ into a subset $\mathbf{L}^* \subseteq P(\mathbf{B})$. Let $\mathbf{L}$ be the smallest lattice with $\mathbf{L}^* \subseteq \mathbf{L}$ with the same operators and ordering relation as for $\mathbf{L}^*$. For the elements of $\mathbf{C}^*$ formal operators $\sqcup$ and $\sqcap$ can be defined and φ^* can be extended to a mapping φ:
>
> $\mathbf{C} = \mathbf{C}^*$ and $\varphi(x) := \varphi^*(x)$ for all $x \in \mathbf{C}^*$,
>
> $\mathbf{C} \leftarrow \mathbf{C} \cup \{x \sqcup y\} \cup \{x \sqcap y\}$ for all $x,y \in \mathbf{C}$,
>
> $\varphi(x \sqcup y) := \varphi(x) \cup \varphi(y)$,
>
> $\varphi(x \sqcap y) := \varphi(x) \cap \varphi(y)$.

If in this formal extension of $\mathbf{C}^*$ the characteristics for the operators $\sqcup$ and $\sqcap$ (Section 3.1.1) are considered, then $\mathbf{C}$ is a lattice with an ordering relation $\leq$, which is defined by $x \sqcap y \leq x$ or $x \leq x \sqcup y$, and $(\mathbf{C},\varphi)$ is a model for $\mathbf{B}$.

Arbitrary relations R_i can be introduced in $\mathbf{C}$, as long as the corresponding relation exists in $\mathbf{L}$. In other words, knowledge concerning $\mathbf{L}$ can be used to define special characteristics in $\mathbf{C}$ (e.g., distributivity). A frequent situation is that the lattice $\mathbf{L}$ shall be described by using a language consisting of words, phrases, and operators with:

- minimum number of words (i.e., elements of $\mathbf{C}^*$ corresponding to an element of $P(\mathbf{B})$),
- possibly simple syntax (i.e., rules for constructing phrases), and
- possibly simple phrases (i.e., elements of $\mathbf{C}$ corresponding to subsets of $P(\mathbf{B})$).

Each rule for constructing phrases corresponds to a rule on the level of sets.

Models can be judged by means of the redundancy introduced in Section 2.2.1.2 through the introduction of a probability distribution over $\mathbf{B}$.

3.2 Basic Formulation of the Classification Problem

We assume a set **B** of n observation units, $\mathbf{B} = \{B_1, B_2, \ldots, B_n\}$, and a set **X** of k attributes, $\mathbf{X} = \{X_1, X_2, \ldots, X_k\}$. Each attribute is defined by a set of values. Then, statistically, the data observed in an observation unit are a realization of the k-dimensional random vector **X** (Table 3.3).

B \ X	X_1	X_2	...	X_k
B_1	x_{11}	x_{12}	...	x_{1k}
B_2	x_{21}	x_{22}	...	x_{2k}
⋮	⋮	⋮	...	⋮
B_n	x_{n1}	x_{n2}	...	x_{nk}

Table 3.3: Matrix of the data x_{ij} observed in n observation units B_i for the k attributes X_j ($i=1,2,\ldots,n$; $j=1,2,\ldots,k$)

In general, we have to allow for missing data, i.e., each attribute has "missing" as one of its values. It may be rational to further classify this value (e.g., as to the cause of missing data, Section 3.1.1).

Classification problems include three types:

(1) Given an attribute or an attribute vector as a dependent variate, we want to investigate the influence of independent attributes on the dependent ones:

- What attributes influence the development of a disease?
- What is the optimal dosage of a drug for the therapy of hypertension?

(2) Given that an observation unit belongs to one out of several populations with known probability distributions of the random vector **X**. We want to assign an observation unit to that population, to which it most probably belongs:

- A patient has symptom cluster **x**. What diagnosis explains it best?
- A patient shall be assigned a diagnosis B_i. In what sequence should we examine the symptoms X_j in order to reach the definite decision as fast as possible (with the most easily obtainable attributes, at minimal costs, ...)?

(3) We assume that an observation unit belongs to one out of several unknown populations. We seek a decomposition of **B** such that observation units in the same subset are as "similar" as possible,

and observation units in different subsets are as "different" as possible:

- A patient has symptom cluster **x**. Is there an error in the data (Section 5.2.2)?
- Classify the diseases (as to diagnostic possibilities, causes, . . .).

The symmetry of **B** and **X** in this fundamental formulation in itself suggests that dual formulations also arise when "attribute" and "observation unit" are exchanged.

The above-listed examples demonstrate the great importance of classification problems. But, because the center of these problems is a more intuitively "defined" concept of similarity, related at least in part to semantic considerations, there is still a lack of satisfying methods for their solution.

In formulating the criteria for judging humans as "similar", anyone experiences how difficult such an explicit formulation of similarity considerations is. In formal algorithmic processing, the human talent for judgement of "gestalt", "form", and "appearence" has to be broken down into simple attributes of different kind. There is no theory defining the important attributes, their values, or the weights these attributes have to be given with respect to their influence on similarity. On the other hand, human judgement has a cost: the variability of the results from different judges and repeated judgements, as well as the impossibility of a reliable ranking, when many objects are to be judged.

The mathematical methods do not have these disadvantages. But it must be kept in mind that mathematical methods have presuppositions rarely accomplished in practice and that results may depend on the selected method itself (Section 3.3.2.2.2).

Certain problems in **decision support** belong to the classification problems.

Because information makes decisions easier or reduces the risk of wrong decisions, every storage and retrieval system is a means for decision support. With a system containing patient data (symptoms, diagnoses, therapies, and outcomes), algorithms may be developed to search for all patients "most similar" to a patient in question. The comparison of the related outcomes will then support a decision about the therapy the new patient should get.

Decision support should not be understood this widely. A decision support should comprise not only data presentation, but also an **algorithm** for making decisions, which can be evaluated and, if necessary, modified by the physician.

This theme has become popular as "computer diagnosis". The term dates from the time when the notion of an "electronic brain" was related to the concept of a machine with practically unlimited capabilities. From this notion many psychologic and social problems arise: the physician's fear of being replaced by a machine, the patient's fear of being confronted with a "mechanized medicine", unsolved problems of responsibility for false decisions, and so on. These problems will not be discussed further. Instead, an introduction into the possibilities and limitations of the methods will be presented, which, because of the complexity of the field, cannot be complete.

The study of algorithms for decision support is useful for the following reasons:

- Algorithms require explicit decision rules. Experience shows, that even experts face serious difficulties in formulating their own rules, and that intensive study improves the basis for the decisions themselves.
- Medicine has become so highly specialized and complicated that diagnostic procedures and therapy frequently require the consultation of experts. But the right expert is not always readily available. A system for decision support may serve to simulate a necessary human expert sufficiently well.
- The utilization of an algorithm for decision support by the physician may have educational functions if the algorithm provides an explanation of its decisions. Furthermore, constant revision to keep the knowledge incorporated into the program up to date may instantly provide medical professionals with state-of-the-art information at all times.

In the following sections, the term "decision" is not restricted to diagnostic problems. The same methods apply to history taking (Section 5.1.3.5), therapy, and prognosis. But in order to avoid using highly abstract terms, uncommon to the physician, the most important methods are explained in the context of diagnosis.

A rough classification of methods may be based on the definition of the diagnostic problem itself. Diagnosis may be interpreted as a "static" conclusion, drawn by mapping a fixed set of symptoms into a fixed set of diagnoses, or - more realistically - as a **process** starting from a certain amount of knowledge and enlarging this amount stepwise until a decision is possible.

For the static interpretation there are several theoretic models available: (1) in special cases, a mathematical function can be formulated (Section 3.3.1.1.2), (2) otherwise a statistical relationship exists (Section 3.3.1.2.1), or (3) a predicate logic model may be found (Section 3.3.1.2.2).

In general, the implementation of a functional dependence is simple. The other two models can be extended to diagnostic processes (Section 3.5), but their strict presuppositions suggest that further models ought to be sought, which are better suited to real situations (Section 3.5.2).

All the methods discussed in the rest of this chapter are, in one way or another, seeking an attribute base for modelling the observation unit (Section 3.1.1).

3.3 Mathematical Classification

The mathematical methods of classification (i.e., the assignment of observation units to populations) are based on the assumption that the k attributes form a k-dimensional **attribute space.** The data are interpreted as points or k-dimensional vectors in this space. Populations correspond to clusters, spreaded over the k-dimensional space. But it is typical of a classification that each population resides in a local subspace. When the clusters are further apart, it is easier to assign the observation unit to the correct population (type I-classification problem, Section 3.3.1.2), or the samples can be more clearly separated (type II-classification problem, Section 3.3.2).

The complexity of the problem increases with the number of dimensions of the attribute space. Therefore, the number of dimensions is tried to be reduced by looking for functional relationships between the attributes (Section 3.3.1.1). Such relationships generate redundancy of the attribute set.

3.3.1 Known Probability Distributions

In this section it is assumed that the populations are known, from which the observation units are drawn. We commonly interpret attributes as **random variables** and formulate the knowledge as **probability distributions.**

3.3.1.1 Dependency Analyses

In mathematical classification dependency analyses are used to reduce the number of dimensions of the attribute space.

If an attribute X_i fully determines another attribute X_j, then the value of X_j has no information when the value of X_i is known for an observation unit. In other words, the observation of X_j is superfluous. For example, the observation of the blood pressure with a Riva-Rocci sphygmomanometer is superfluous when data are available from intraarterial measurements.

Because the data contain random errors, the above-mentioned case is unrealistic. Instead, the relation may be modelled by the regression function

$$X_j = f(X_i) + E,$$

interpreting the attribute X_j as a sum of a deterministic function f of X_i and of a random error E. Complex dependences exist when the attribute X_j depends on a combination of attributes or when a combination of attributes depends on a combination of other attributes.

The results of a dependency analysis should be interpreted with caution. Errors usually arise when a statistically demonstrated relationship is interpreted as **causal**. In addition to the causal relation, which is certainly of prime practical interest, there are other possibilities. Two variables may both depend on another variable which has been overlooked, or variables may merely be formally related (e.g., two random variables whose sum is a constant).

A reduction of the attribute space corresponds to a transformation of the observation matrix (Table 3.3) into a matrix with less than k columns, or to a transformation of the attributes X_i $(i=1,2,\ldots,k_x)$ into attributes Y_j $(j=1,2,\ldots,k_y)$ with $k_y < k_x$. In general, these transformations cause a loss of information.

Simple transformations consist of dropping certain attributes. This corresponds to a projection of the attribute space into a space of lesser dimension **(attribute selection)**. Obviously, the attributes dropped should be those, which depend on other attributes to a high degree, or those with values more or less constant in the set of observation units.

3.3.1.1.1 Dependency Measures

The **correlation coefficient** is a measure of the relationship between two random variables. The **multiple** correlation coefficient of random variable Y with respect to a set $\{X_1, X_2, \ldots, X_m\}$ of random variables is a measure for the dependence of Y on this set. **Partial** correlation coefficients are correlation coefficients between two random variables of a conditional multivariate distribution [93].

3.3.1.1.2 Dependence of Dependent Variates on Independent Variates

The statistical analysis of a relation between a set of dependent variates and a set of independent variates is most fully developed in the **linear model**:

$$\mathbf{Y} = \mathbf{X}'\cdot\mathbf{B} + \mathbf{F}'\cdot\Gamma + \mathbf{E}.$$

$\mathbf{Y}$ is a matrix of dependent random variables, $\mathbf{X}$ is a matrix of continuous independent variates (**covariates**), $\mathbf{B}$ is a matrix of regression coefficients, $\mathbf{F}$ is a matrix of non-continuous independent variates (**factors**) fixed by the model, Γ is a matrix of "effects", and $\mathbf{E}$ is a matrix of random errors. The errors are presumed to follow a multivariate normal distribution.

If $\mathbf{F}=\mathbf{0}$, then the problem is one of **regression analysis**. If $\mathbf{X}=\mathbf{0}$, then the problem refers to **analysis of variance**. If neither $\mathbf{X}$ nor $\mathbf{F}$ are $\mathbf{0}$, then the problem becomes one of **analysis of covariance**. The reader is referred to the special literature for a more detailed description of these methods [9,56,140].

At present, in only a few cases is the relation between diagnosis and therapy so well-known that it can be described by means of mathematical functions.

One-sided aphakia due to a grey cataract usually remains uncorrected by a one-sided cataract lens because of the different sizes of the two images, if the other eye still has sufficient sight. In such cases, contact lenses also result in different sizes of the images. The development of ultrasound measuring methods has recently made the determination of sizes and refractions so exact that combined correction is possible, which retains binocular sight [51].

Another example is electrolyte- or acid-base balance. The relation between blood-pH, on the one hand, and kidney function and electrolyte concentration, on the other hand, can be described adequately by mathematical functions [16]. Furthermore, exact recording of intake and excretion of fluids and electrolytes provides an adequate guide to the physician in therapy [44].

Simulation methods are successfully employed in planning and administration of certain therapies. They are based on a mathematical model of the effect of a drug depending on dosage and specific patient-oriented attributes. Such models not only use clinical experience, but also the results of pharmacological or physical tests. Decision support is especially important for drugs having a small therapeutic margin of safety for dosage, administration method, or administration time.

Examples are therapies with digitalis [75], antiepileptics, antibiotics, lithium, cytostatic drugs, antiarrhythmic drugs, insulin [20], anticoagulants [166], or ionizing radiation (Section 6.1.4).

3.3.1.1.3 Correlations Between Components of a Random Vector

Principal component analysis looks for a sequence of linear transformations of a standardized random vector $\mathbf{x}$ with the following characteristics:

We choose a vector β with $|\beta| = 1$ such that the variance of $\beta'\cdot\mathbf{x}$ is maximized (Σ = covariance matrix of $\mathbf{x}$):

$$E\left((\beta'\cdot\mathbf{x})^2\right) = E(\beta'\cdot\mathbf{x}\cdot\mathbf{x}'\cdot\beta) = E(\beta'\cdot\Sigma\cdot\beta) = \max .$$

From well-known theorems of linear algebra, β is a solution of the following eigenvalue-problem:

$$(\Sigma - \lambda\cdot\mathbf{I})\cdot\beta = 0 \qquad (\mathbb{I} = \text{unity matrix}) .$$

The maximum condition corresponds to the condition that β is the eigenvector corresponding to the greatest eigenvalue λ. After determination of β a further linear transformation $\beta'^{(1)}\cdot\mathbf{x}$ is sought with $|\beta^{(1)}|=1$, $\beta'\cdot\mathbf{x}$ and $\beta'^{(1)}\cdot\mathbf{x}$ independent, and variance of $\beta'^{(1)}\cdot\mathbf{x}$ maximal.

These transformations are repeated as long as there are solutions of the eigenvalue-problem. The method corresponds geometrically to a **rotation** of the coordinate system such that the axes are orthogonal and variance is maximal in each direction. The primary objective is a transformation of the random vector into a space of lesser dimension, i.e., an explanation of the variation of the data by a few independent linear combinations of the original random variables.

Principal component analysis is a specialization of **factor analysis.** In factor analysis, the coordinate system is rotated such that "factors" are created, which may be interpreted as clearly as possible, and which explain most of the variance.

Canonical analysis has a similar objective. From a random vector $\mathbf{x}$, consisting of two parts $\mathbf{x}' = (\mathbf{x}'^{(1)}, \mathbf{x}'^{(2)})$, we seek a linear transformation,

$$U = \alpha' \cdot \mathbf{x}^{(1)}, \quad V = \beta' \cdot \mathbf{x}^{(2)},$$

such that U and V are maximally correlated. The transformation is repeated,

$$U^{(1)} = \alpha'^{(1)} \cdot \mathbf{x}^{(1)}, \quad V^{(1)} = \beta'^{(1)} \cdot \mathbf{x}^{(2)},$$

such that U and $U^{(1)}$ as well as V and $V^{(1)}$ are independent, and $U^{(1)}$ and $V^{(1)}$ are maximally correlated. Again, this method results in an eigenvalue-problem. It corresponds to a transformation of the subspaces of $\mathbf{x}^{(1)}$ and $\mathbf{x}^{(2)}$ into orthogonal subspaces such that the related "canonical" variables are maximally dependent.

3.3.1.1.4 Contingency-Table Analysis

We take up the case of two attributes X and Y only. The formulas for the theoretically simple generalization to more than two attributes may be taken from the more specific literature.

Let continuous attributes be classified. n observation units are drawn having one of the levels $(x_1^*, x_2^*, \ldots, x_k^*)$ of attribute X and one of the levels $(y_1^*, y_2^*, \ldots, y_\ell^*)$ of attribute Y. The frequencies N_{ij} of the combinations (x_i^*, y_j^*) are arranged in a **contingemcy-table** (Table 3.4).

X \ Y	y_1^*	...	y_j^*	...	y_ℓ^*	Sum of rows
x_1^*	N_{11}	...	N_{1j}	...	$N_{1\ell}$	$N_{1\bullet}$
⋮	⋮		⋮		⋮	⋮
x_i^*	N_{i1}	...	N_{ij}	...	$N_{i\ell}$	$N_{i\bullet}$
⋮	⋮		⋮		⋮	⋮
x_k^*	N_{k1}	...	N_{kj}	...	$N_{k\ell}$	$N_{k\bullet}$
Sum of columns	$N_{\bullet 1}$	...	$N_{\bullet j}$	...	$N_{\bullet \ell}$	n

Table 3.4: Contingency-table for the data of attributes X and Y

If the **marginal probabilities** $p_{i\cdot}$ for the level x_i^* and $p_{\cdot j}$ for the level y_j^* are known and if X and Y are independent, then the expectation for the **occupation frequency** N_{ij} is from (2.2)

$$(3.1) \qquad E(N_{ij}) = n \cdot p_{i\cdot} \cdot p_{\cdot j},$$

and the test statistic

$$\chi^2 = \sum_{i=1}^{k} \sum_{j=1}^{\ell} \frac{\left[N_{ij} - E(N_{ij})\right]^2}{E(N_{ij})}$$

has an approximate $\chi^2_{k\cdot\ell-1}$-distribution [85].

3.3.1.2 Assignment to a Population Type I-Classification Problem

3.3.1.2.1 Statistical Decision Models

Several attributes are observed in a randomly drawn observation unit. On the basis of these data the observation unit is to be assigned to a population. There is a finite set of populations, each one described by a multivariate distribution of the random vector.

If there are two populations V_1 and V_2, then there are four possibilities (Table 3.5).

		True population V_1	True population V_2
Assigned population	V_1	0	K(1|2)
Assigned population	V_2	K(2|1)	0

Table 3.5: Costs of assigning an observation unit to one of two populations V_1 and V_2

Let V_1 be the population of "healthy" people and V_2 the population of people with "uremia". The populations are described by the respective density function of the continuous attribute X = "serum urea" (Fig. 3.5). The value of X is observed in a "patient". We have to decide whether he is healthy or sick.

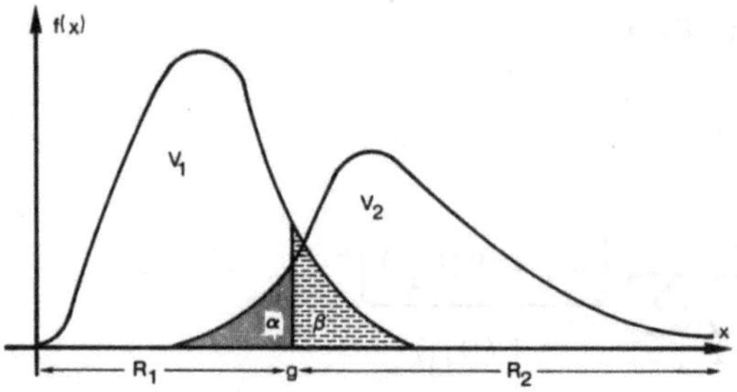

Fig. 3.5: Schema of the probability densities for a continuous attribute X in two populations V_1 and V_2

Then the strategy $R = (R_1,R_2)$ for assignment to one of the two populations is defined as: if the datum $x \in R_1$, then the "patient" is classified as healthy; otherwise as sick.

No matter where the boundary g is located, a healthy patient will be classified as sick with probability β and a sick patient will be classified as healthy with probability α. Each choice of the boundary g partitions the x-axis into two parts R_1 and R_2. If we let the costs of classifying a sick patient as healthy be 5 units, the costs of classifying a healthy patient as sick be 3 units, and the (a priori-)probability that the patient is healthy be p, then the expected costs of the strategy R are

$$p \cdot 3 \cdot \beta + (1-p) \cdot 5 \cdot \alpha \, .$$

Now we wish to minimize the costs by determining the strategy R, i.e., the boundary g, such that the expected costs are minimized. If $f_1(x)$ and $f_2(x)$ are the respective probability densities, then g has to be determined such that

$$p \cdot 3 \cdot \underbrace{\int_{g}^{\infty} f_1(x)\,dx}_{\beta} + (1-p) \cdot 5 \cdot \underbrace{\int_{-\infty}^{g} f_2(x)\,dx}_{\alpha}$$

is minimized.

A **decision strategy** should be such that the probability of a false decision is minimized. If the "costs" of both false decisions differ, i.e., the costs $K(1|2)$ of a decision for V_1 if V_2 is correct differs from the costs $K(2|1)$ of a decision for V_2 if V_1 is correct, then the "mean" costs of the strategy should be minimized.

The vector $\mathbf{x}=(x_1,x_2,\ldots,x_k)$ is interpreted as a point in a k-dimensional space. Now, a decision strategy $R=(R_1,R_2)$ is such that the k-dimensional space R is partitioned into two subspaces R_1 and R_2. If the point $\mathbf{x}$ is located in R_i, then the observation unit is assigned to population V_i (i=1,2).

The expected **costs** of a false assignment are:

$$(3.2)\qquad \begin{Bmatrix} k(1,R) = K(2|1)\cdot P(\mathbf{x}\in R_2|\mathbf{x}\in V_1) \text{ if assigned to } V_2 \\ k(2,R) = K(1|2)\cdot P(\mathbf{x}\in R_1|\mathbf{x}\in V_2) \text{ if assigned to } V_1 \end{Bmatrix}.$$

If the a priori-probability p for drawing an observation unit from V_1 is known, then the expected total costs of strategy R are equal to

$$p\cdot k(1,R) + (1-p)\cdot k(2,R)\ .$$

A reasonable principle for the selection of a strategy in this case is the minimization of the expected total costs (**BAYES procedure**) [155]. Thus, a BAYES procedure minimizes the expression

$$(3.3)\qquad c\cdot k(1,R) + k(2,R)\quad ,\quad c = \frac{p}{1-p} > 0.$$

When p is unknown, the **minimax**-principle may be used; the requested procedure should be such that

$$\min_R \max \Big(k(1,R),k(2,R)\Big).$$

A strategy R is at least as **good** as a strategy S, if

$$k(i,R) \le k(i,S)\qquad (i=1,2).$$

R is **better** than S if at least in one inequality the equal sign is omitted. A strategy is **admissable** if there is no better strategy.

If p is unknown, then the set of all admissable strategies consists of all BAYES procedures [9].

Let be $f_i(\mathbf{x})$ the density of the random vector $\mathbf{x}$ in the population V_i (i=1,2). Then from (3.2) and (3.3) the expected total costs are:

$$c\cdot K(2|1)\cdot \int_{R_2} f_1(\mathbf{x})d\mathbf{x} + K(1|2)\cdot \int_{R_1} f_2(\mathbf{x})d\mathbf{x}.$$

Because R_1 and R_2 are disjoint, it follows

$$\int_{R_2}\left(c\cdot K(2|1)\cdot f_1(\mathbf{x}) - K(1|2)\cdot f_2(\mathbf{x})\right)d\mathbf{x} + K(1|2)\cdot \underbrace{\int_{R_1\cup R_2} f_2(\mathbf{x})\,d\mathbf{x}}_{1} \quad .$$

Thus, the expected total costs are minimized if R_2 is chosen such that it contains exactly those points $\mathbf{x}$, for which

$$c\cdot K(2|1)\cdot f_1(\mathbf{x}) - K(1|2)\cdot f_2(\mathbf{x}) < 0 \; .$$

Therefore, the optimal strategy is defined by

$$\left\{\begin{array}{l} R_1 \; : \; \dfrac{f_1(\mathbf{x})}{f_2(\mathbf{x})} \geq \dfrac{K(1|2)}{c\cdot K(2|1)} \\ \\ R_2 \; : \; \text{otherwise} \end{array}\right\} \quad .$$

This strategy can be generalized for the classification problem with m populations:

If p_i $(i=1,2,\ldots,m)$ is the a priori-probability for drawing an observation unit B from population V_i with the density $f_i(\mathbf{x})$, and if $K(j|i)$ are the costs of assignment to population V_j, then the partitioning $\{R_1,R_2,\ldots,R_m\}$ minimizing the expected total costs is defined by the following rule:

Assign the observation unit to that population V_k, for which

$$\sum_{\substack{i=1\\ i\neq k}}^{m} p_i\cdot f_i(\mathbf{x})\cdot K(k|i), \quad p_i = P(B \in V_i), \quad f_i(\mathbf{x}) = P(\mathbf{X}=\mathbf{x}|B \in V_i)$$

is minimal $(k=1,2,\ldots,m)$.

Because $f_i(\mathbf{x})$ is the conditional probability (density) that an observation unit from V_i has attribute vector $\mathbf{x}$, from (2.1) the product $p_i\cdot f_i(\mathbf{x})$ is the probability (density) that an observation unit is from V_i **and** has attribute vector $\mathbf{x}$.

If the costs $K(j|i)$ of a false assignment of an element from V_i to V_j are all equal, and if the populations V_i are a decomposition, then the rule may be formulated as follows:

Assign the observation unit to that population V_k, for which

$$\sum_{\substack{i=1\\i\neq k}}^{m} p_i \cdot f_i(\mathbf{x}) = \sum_{i=1}^{m} p_i \cdot f_i(\mathbf{x}) - p_k \cdot f_k(\mathbf{x})$$

is minimal, or for which $p_k \cdot f_k(\mathbf{x})$ is maximal $(k=1,2,\ldots,m)$.

This likelihood solution is directly perceived:

An observation unit is assigned to that population, for which the probability that it is drawn from this population **and** has attribute vector $\mathbf{x}$ is maximal.

This formulation also clearly reveals the relation to the BAYES theorem [85] and the statistical decision model based on it (Section 3.5.2.1).

Discriminant analysis [91] uses another criterion for optimization. The fundamental idea is explained by a 2-dimensional example.

Fig. 3.6 contains two clusters corresponding to samples from two populations with the 2-dimensional densities $f_1(\mathbf{x})$ and $f_2(\mathbf{x})$, $\mathbf{x}=(x_1,x_2)$. A new axis y_1 is computed that separates the samples "as well as possible". The ratio of the variance between the samples and the variance within the samples is used as measure of the degree of separation. This ratio is minimized depending on the linear transformation leading to axis y_1. Then a second axis y_2 is computed, which must be orthogonal to y_1, following the same criterion (in the 2-dimensional case, y_2 is determined by y_1).

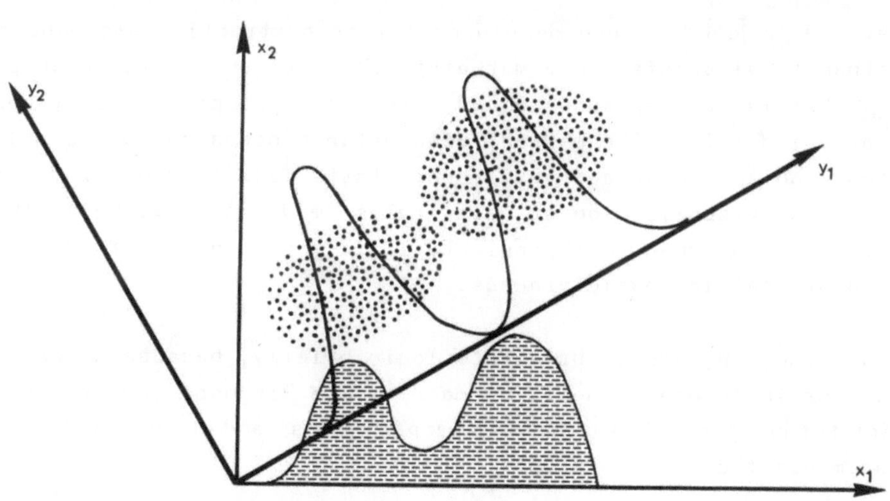

Fig. 3.6: Schema of two samples and of the probability densities on different axes

If the distributions are multivariate normal with identical covariance matrices, then both methods result in the same strategies. There is a test for this special case, which may be used to determine the number of discriminant functions necessary for explaining the total variance. Unknown expectations and covariance matrix can be estimated from the samples [9].

The method is also applicable to discrete random variables.

Given two populations V_1 and V_2 and two random variables X_1 and X_2 with the values x^*_{11}, x^*_{12}, and x^*_{21}, x^*_{22}, respectively. Assume probabilities:

X_1 \ X_2	x^*_{21}	x^*_{22}
x^*_{11}	1/4	1/4
x^*_{12}	1/4	1/4

for V_1,

X_1 \ X_2	x^*_{21}	x^*_{22}
x^*_{11}	1/8	1/4
x^*_{12}	1/8	1/2

for V_2.

Then, for equal a priori-probabilities and equal costs of a false assignment, the optimal strategy $R = (R_1, R_2)$ is defined by $R_1 = \{(x^*_{11}, x^*_{21}), (x^*_{11}, x^*_{22}), (x^*_{12}, x^*_{21})\}$ and $R_2 = \{(x^*_{12}, x^*_{22})\}$.

3.3.1.2.2 Predicate Logic Decision Model

Predicate logic [65] has been developed for reconstructing and understanding mathematical proofs. In a mathematical proof one starts with propositions (axioms, assumptions) and derives other propositions by application of valid rules. The medical diagnostic process may be formulated analogously on this abstract level: one starts from findings and derives the diagnosis by application of valid rules (medical knowledge). Therefore, it can be assumed that predicate logic may furnish a formal description of the diagnostic process.

We explain the language of predicate logic briefly, because it has had an important influence on decision models. The language consists of elements for formulation of statements (propositions) and rules for deducing new statements from previous ones.

Constants are objects, which may be given an identifying name (e.g., LIVER).

Variables stand for different objects at different times.

Predicates denote properties. For example, the property that the liver is an organ can be expressed by a predicate: ORGAN(LIVER). The **value** of a predicate is "true" or "false", i.e., whether or not the constant argument LIVER has the property ORGAN. Predicates can have more than one argument. For example, the fact that diabetes is a risk during pregnancy can be expressed by a two-place predicate

RISK(DIABETES, PREGNANCY).

The "solution" of a predicate is a **statement** ("Diabetes is a risk during pregnancy").

The values "true" and "false" are usually denoted by "1" and "0".

Functions have arguments, like predicates, and result in a value (not a truth-value). For example, the function CONSISTENCY with the argument LIVER may have the values COARSE and SOFT. Functions may be arguments of predicates but not vice versa.

The fundamental function type for an **object triplet** (Section 3.1.3) is

VALUE(OBSERVATION UNIT,ATTRIBUTE).

Operators operate on one (negation) or two predicates (conjunction, disjunction, implication) (Fig. 3.7). They are used for formulating **expressions**. To formulate the concept that the liver is coarse and enlarged, the following expression is formed:

COARSENESS(CONSISTENCY(LIVER)) $\wedge$ ENLARGEMENT(LIVER) .

It consists of two predicates, COARSENESS and ENLARGEMENT, which are connected by the operator $\wedge$. The argument of the predicate COARSENESS is the value of the function CONSISTENCY for the argument LIVER.

Quantifiers also occur in the formulation of expressions. To express the observation that **all** tests t from a defined set T have a normal result, the universal quantifier "for all" is used (denoted by $\forall$):

$\forall(t \in T)$ (RESULT(t) = NORMAL) .

If there is **at least one** test with a normal result, then the existential quantifier "there is" is used (denoted by $\exists$):

$\exists(t \in T)$ (RESULT(t) = NORMAL) .

Given a problem with two symptoms s_1 and s_2 and two diagnoses d_1 and d_2; for simplicity, the symptoms and diagnoses are formulated as predicates themselves (x is a patient variable):

$s_1(x)$, $s_2(x)$, $d_1(x)$, $d_2(x)$.

We assume two rules for the applicable medical knowledge:

(1) If symptom s_1 is present, then disease d_2 is present ($s_1 \rightarrow d_2$).

(2) If symptom s_2 is present, then disease d_1 is not present ($s_2 \rightarrow \bar{d}_1$).

ℓ_1	ℓ_2	"not" ℓ_1	ℓ_1 "and" ℓ_2	ℓ_1 "or" ℓ_2	"if" ℓ_1 "then" ℓ_2
1	1	0	1	1	1
1	0	0	0	1	0
0	1	1	0	1	1
0	0	1	0	0	1
		Negation	Conjunction	Disjunction	Implication

Fig. 3.7: Truth tables for the logical operators with predicates ℓ_1 and ℓ_2 (1: true, 0: false)

A patient a may have symptom s_1 (i.e., $s_1(a)=1$). From this finding, we deduce all possible valid statements concerning the diagnoses. This means that each of the statements concerning diagnoses, $\{d_1(a)=1,\ d_1(a)=0,\ d_2(a)=1,\ d_2(a)=0\}$, has to be tested for consistency with both the specific finding and the medical knowledge, integrating both of these into total knowledge W:

$$W = s_1 \wedge \left((s_1 \longrightarrow d_2) \wedge (s_2 \longrightarrow \bar{d}_1)\right).$$

Because $\ell_1 \longrightarrow \ell_2$ and $\bar{\ell}_1 \vee \ell_2$ are equivalent, this equation is equivalent to

$$W = s_1 \wedge \left((\bar{s}_1 \vee d_2) \wedge (\bar{s}_2 \vee \bar{d}_1)\right) = \left(\underbrace{(s_1 \wedge \bar{s}_1)}_{0} \vee (s_1 \wedge d_2)\right) \wedge (\bar{s}_2 \vee \bar{d}_1) = s_1 \wedge d_2 \wedge (\bar{s}_2 \vee \bar{d}_1).$$

Because $s_1 = 1$, this is equivalent to

$$W = d_2 \wedge (\bar{s}_2 \vee \bar{d}_1).$$

Because the specific finding and the medical knowledge have to be consistent, W must have the value 1. This is only possible if d_2 has value 1. From this it follows that d_2 is a correct diagnosis. Nothing can be deduced for d_1, because s_2 is unknown.

3.3.2 Classification of an Observation Unit Type II-Classification Problem

The type II-classification problem is characterized by a sample **B** of n observation units, described by an attribute vector $\mathbf{X}=(X_1,X_2,\ldots,X_k)$.

The elements of the sample are assumed to be drawn from different populations. The sample is to be decomposed into subsets (**classes**) such that (1) elements from the same class are as homogeneous as possible and (2) elements from different classes are as inhomogeneous as possible. These two postulations are interrelated. The problem is degenerate when the number of populations is not smaller than the sample size, because there is always the trivial solution of one class for each observation unit.

The observation units can be interpreted as points in a k-dimensional space formed by the attributes of vector **X**. A "good" decomposition is possible when subsets can be found in separate parts of the space (Fig. 3.8).

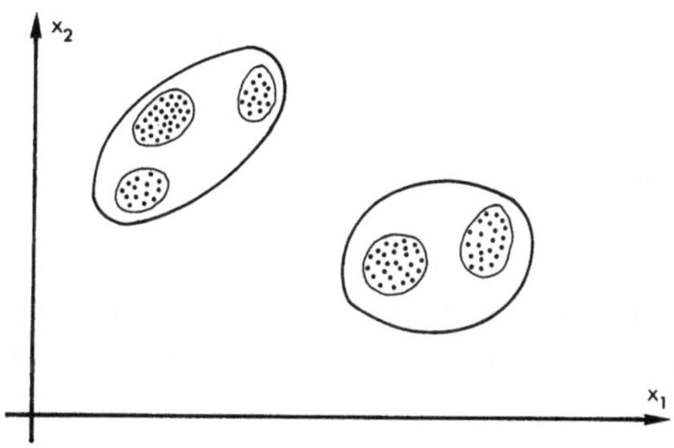

Fig. 3.8: Decomposition of a 2-dimensional scatter diagram

The type II-classification problem is frequently based on the idea of a "natural" order of the observation units, which must be extracted from multiple attributes. Basically, the procedure seeks to find an attribute base (Section 3.1.1) by starting from a "semantically" defined attribute set, applying formal transformations based on a quantitative attribute ("distance"), and hopefully arriving at an attribute set reflecting a natural order. But, because the natural relations among the attributes are unknown, such classifications are largely subjective, even if "objective" methods are applied. This subjectivity is derived from the selection of attributes, the similarity/distance measure, and the algorithm. In spite of this deficiency, the mathematical methods of classification have a great advantage in that they can be reviewed and repeated, in contrast to a pure judgement by experts, which cannot.

A type II-classification problem may also be illustrated by the following interpretation: A close examination of a sample gives a more distinct view of the individual elements. If one looks at the sample from a greater distance, then the small differences among elements disappear, and eventually some elements merge and clusters of elements are recognized. Depending on the arrangement of the individual elements, this process can be repeated on different levels (for example, note the different information in a newspaper picture seen from a normal distance and through a magnifying glass).

Neglect of "small" differences corresponds to an increase of redundancy (Section 2.2.1.2). This principle is fundamental in all methods of **cluster analysis** or pattern recognition, alternate names for the type II-classification problem.

The simplest case is the definition of a class by a set of values (e.g., all points falling into a hyperplane of the attribute space). If continuous attributes are included, then intervals may also be used (for example, if there are two continuous attributes and one discrete attribute, then a class may be defined such that it contains all elements with the same level of the discrete attribute).

In a few special situations factor analysis may be applied.

The type II-classification problem is often reduced to type I by estimating the necessary probability distributions, using the respective frequency distributions from a "training set", and afterwards classifying the actual "test set".

3.3.2.1 Configuration-Frequency Analysis

The method described in Section 3.3.1.1.4 can also be applied to the type II-classification problem. Unknown marginal probabilities may be estimated from the sample. The estimation of the expectation (3.1) is:

$$N^*_{ij} = \frac{N_{i.} \cdot N_{.j}}{n} .$$

Then, the test statistic

$$\chi^2 = \sum_{i=1}^{k} \sum_{j=1}^{\ell} \frac{(N_{ij} - N^*_{ij})^2}{N^*_{ij}}$$

has an approximate $\chi^2_{(k-1)\cdot(\ell-1)}$-distribution.

In a **hierarchic** configuration-frequency analysis for the construction of a hierarchic classification, all contingency-tables with t out of the k attributes ($t=k,k-1,\ldots,2$) are computed, and the contingency-table with the "most significant" χ^2 is investigated further. Because simultaneous tests have to be made, the error probability has to be adjusted [88].

3.3.2.2 Cluster Analysis

3.3.2.2.1 Distance/Similarity

Cluster analysis [108] comprises a set of methods, all leading to the construction of classes by neglecting "small" differences and thus increasing redundancy (Section 2.2.1.2). These methods are all based on the definition of a "distance" (or "similarity") among elements. The intuitive concept of similarity reflects the idea that elements are more similar if they differ "not much" with respect to "important" attributes. Because "distance" and "similarity" are complementary concepts, we employ the concept of "distance" in the following discussion.

In order to treat the problem by mathematical means, the following assumptions are required:

- distance function for observation units,
  - attributes (independent variates) for computation of the distance,
  - effect of an attribute on the distance,
- distance function for classes (sets).

The distance function for classes must be specifically defined, if the nesting of classes is required.

The **distance function** $f(\mathbf{X},\mathbf{Y})$ for two arbitrary points $\mathbf{X}$ and $\mathbf{Y}$ in a k-dimensional space is essentially real-valued. Appropriate requirements for such functions are:

$f(\mathbf{X},\mathbf{Y}) \geq 0$	(distance is a non-negative number),
$f(\mathbf{X},\mathbf{Y}) > 0 \rightleftarrows \mathbf{X} \neq \mathbf{Y}$	(two different observation units have always a positive distance),
$f(\mathbf{X},\mathbf{Y}) = f(\mathbf{Y},\mathbf{X})$	(distance is symmetric).

A **metric** is a distance function, for which the triangle inequality holds (distance from **X** to **Y** to **Z** is at least as great as the direct distance from **X** to **Z**):

$$f(\mathbf{X},\mathbf{Y}) + f(\mathbf{Y},\mathbf{Z}) \geq f(\mathbf{X},\mathbf{Z}).$$

A **similarity function** $g(\mathbf{X},\mathbf{Y})$ may be defined analogously.

If distance and similarity are normalized to the range $[0,1]$, then the similarity function can directly be derived from a distance function. For example, such a definition is:

$$g(\mathbf{X},\mathbf{Y}) = 1 - f(\mathbf{X},\mathbf{Y}) .$$

In this definition $g=1$ corresponds to maximum similarity and $g=0$ corresponds to minimum similarity.

Difficulties arise in practical situations particularly when qualitative attributes are included and data are missing. It is impossible to state general rules for handling these problems. The problem of qualitative attributes, for which a mean is not defined, is bypassed formally by the introduction of random variables, i.e., by numerical coding of the qualitative data. The interpretation of the distance in such cases depends on the specific application. In case of missing data, we often omit from the sample the respective observation units. Missing quantitative data are sometimes replaced by the corresponding mean, restricting the interpretation as above. It is always possible to treat each attribute in the same way by "reduction" of the attributes to the highest possible level (e.g., the classification of continuous attributes leads to "discrete" attributes). This procedure always results in loss of information, which may not be tolerable.

3.3.2.2.1.1 Qualitative Attributes

A simple class of distance functions, which is often used, is based on the interpretation of a row vector of the observation matrix (Table 3.3 in Section 3.2) as a character string. Given the character strings:

$$\mathbf{X} = x_1\, x_2 \ldots x_k$$

$$\mathbf{Y} = y_1\, y_2 \ldots y_k .$$

If the original lengths are different, then the shorter string can be filled with the empty character. The **HAMMING distance** h is the number of positions where **X** and **Y** differ:

$$h = \sum_{i=1}^{k} \delta_i , \quad \delta_i = \begin{cases} 0, & x_i = y_i \\ 1, & \text{otherwise} \end{cases} .$$

The HAMMING distance between EXANTHEMAS and ENANTHEMA is equal to 2.

This distance can be normalized by use of the **relative HAMMING distance**

$$H = \frac{h}{k} .$$

It is a metric with the same weight for each attribute.

Taking the intuitive idea as a basis, then it seems reasonable to use the HAMMING distance as long as there is no additional knowledge concerning the attributes and their relations. There are various modifications of this distance, which one gets by introducing weights:

$$h = \sum_{i=1}^{k} g_i \cdot \delta_i .$$

Because weights have a great influence on the distance, they should be used only when they are sufficiently well-founded on the problem. For example, meaningful weights can be deduced from the measures of "trustworthiness" (Section 3.1.3 and [154]).

3.3.2.2.1.2 Quantitative Attributes

The most important class of distance functions are the **L_r-distances**:

$$L_r(\mathbf{X},\mathbf{Y}) = \left(\sum_{i=1}^{k} |x_i - y_i|^r \right)^{1/r} , \quad r > 0.$$

With increasing r, the influence of attributes with a great range increases. The L_r-distances are invariant for translation of the coordinate system but depend on scale. Therefore, the random variables should be

standardized. This transformation is performed by subtracting the expectation μ_i from the random variable X_i and dividing the difference by the standard deviation σ_i:

$$Z_i = \frac{X_i - \mu_i}{\sigma_i} \quad .$$

The standardized random variables Z_i have expectation 0 and standard deviation 1. The corresponding standardized data are equal to the deviation from the mean, measured in units of the empirical standard deviation.

Two frequently used special cases of the L_r-distances are the sum (or mean) of the distances of the components (r=1) and the Euclidean distance (r=2). The latter is invariant for rotation of the coordinate system.

The **MAHALANOBIS distance**

$$f(\mathbf{X},\mathbf{Y}) = \sqrt{(\mathbf{X}-\mathbf{Y})' \cdot \Sigma^{-1} \cdot (\mathbf{X}-\mathbf{Y})} \quad , \quad \Sigma = \text{covariance matrix},$$

is invariant for translation, rotation, and change of scale. In addition, it considers the effect of correlations among the attributes. If the covariance matrix is neglected, then the MAHALANOBIS distance leads to the Euclidean distance.

3.3.2.2.1.3 Classes

Distance functions for classes are based on the distance function for elements.

Let $\mathbf{B}_1$ and $\mathbf{B}_2$ be two classes of observation units with the sizes n_1 and n_2, respectively. A distance function $f_{\mathbf{XY}} = f(\mathbf{X},\mathbf{Y})$ is to be defined for elements ($\mathbf{X} \in \mathbf{B}_1$, $\mathbf{Y} \in \mathbf{B}_2$).

The most important distance functions between classes are:

1) $F_{12} = \min_{\mathbf{X},\mathbf{Y}} f_{\mathbf{XY}}$ Single linkage.

2) $F_{12} = \frac{1}{n_1 \cdot n_2} \cdot \sum_{\mathbf{X},\mathbf{Y}} f_{\mathbf{XY}}$ Average linkage.

3) $F_{12} = \max_{\mathbf{X},\mathbf{Y}} f_{\mathbf{XY}}$ Complete linkage.

4) $F_{12} = \sqrt{(\bar{\mathbf{X}} - \bar{\mathbf{Y}})' \cdot \mathbf{\Sigma}^{-1} \cdot (\bar{\mathbf{X}} - \bar{\mathbf{Y}})}$ MAHALANOBIS distance.

This MAHALANOBIS distance essentially determines the confidence limits of the difference between the mean vectors of two multivariate normal distributed populations ($\mathbf{\Sigma}$ = covariance matrix).

5) $F_{12} = |\bar{\mathbf{X}} - \bar{\mathbf{Y}}| = L_2(\bar{\mathbf{X}},\bar{\mathbf{Y}})$ Euclidean distance.

Euclidean distance between the mean vectors of both samples. This distance results from the MAHALANOBIS distance by neglecting the covariance matrix.

The distances 4) and 5) require quantitative attributes. The distances 2) to 5) generate "compact", spheric classes. The distance 1) may generate diffuse, long-drawn-out classes, if there are "bridges" between classes.

3.3.2.2.2 <u>Algorithms</u>

We omit a detailed presentation of algorithms, widely available in the more specific literature [156,192], but include the essential principles. For a theoretic background the reader is referred to Section 3.1.

For **hierarchic** classification, the following approach can be used:

The n observation units form 1-element classes (level 0). Level t comprises (n-t) classes (t=0,1,...,n-1): $C_1, C_2, \ldots, C_{n-t}$. For each level the two classes C_i and C_j with minimum distance are united (Section 3.3.2.2.1.3) to form level (t+1). The procedure is repeated until every element is included in the same class. This leads to a hierarchic structure (**dendrogram**) with the individual observation units on the lowest level and the set of all observation units on the highest level (Fig. 3.9).

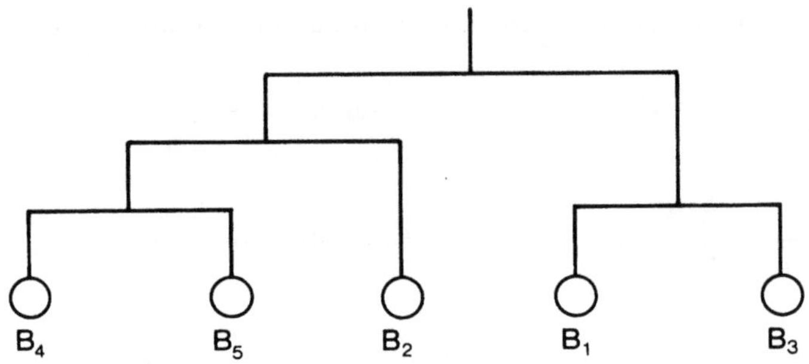

Fig. 3.9: Dendrogram in hierarchic classification of the observation units B_1 to B_5

A typical algorithm for **nom-hierarchic** classification is:

Assume a number $d \geq 0$. Starting from an arbitrary observation unit B_i form a class comprising all observation units located in the d-environment of B_i (i.e., whose distance is not greater than d). In the next step each observation unit is included in the class, which lies in the d-environment of at least one member of the class. The class is complete when all elements in the d-environment of at least one element are included in the class. Starting from an arbitrary element outside the class the next class is constructed according to the same procedure.

Certain classes emerge from this procedure, within which each element has at least one neighbor in its d-environment and is more than d distant from all outside elements. Therefore, the result is independent of the order of the constructing process. However, the classes depend strongly on the value of d. If $d=0$, then only 1-element classes result; if $d \rightarrow \infty$, then all elements fall in the same class.

The method can also be applied to hierarchic classification. In this case, one starts with $d=0$ and increases d stepwise.

Cluster analysis depends strongly on the particular method; the result must, therefore, be interpreted very cautiously. The following criteria for cluster analysis have been postulated [154]:

(1) The information content of a class should be as high as possible and should be based on as many attributes as possible.

(2) Each attribute should be equally weighted.

(3) Similarity between two observation units should be related to all attributes.

These postulations seem plausible, but they can hardly be realized in practice. Thus (2) is equivalent to a uniform effect of the differences among values of different attributes on the distance. Therefore, in some methods attributes with a large range effect the distance more than attributes with a low range. Restriction to quantitative attributes makes the analysis easier. Thus, the MAHALANOBIS distance considers not only differences in expectations and variances, but also correlations between attributes. However, there is no "natural" comparison among different values of qualitative and quantitative attributes. This problem is not solved by the reduction of attributes (for example, by dichotomizing quantitative attributes, Section 3.1.2).

Construction of higher level classes by computing the distances between lower level classes is an optimal procedure when an a priori-classification exists. However, in such a case these methods are not needed. Cluster analysis does not prove a natural classification, but is at best suited for hypothesis generation. The utility has to be checked by considering how well the classification meets its purposes.

3.4 Classification of Concepts

This section deals with classifications, for which observation units are **concepts**. If the construction of a model for a domain and for its information content is formulated on the highly abstract level of Section 3.2, then a special section may not seem to be justified. However, the practical significance of this kind of analysis, the volume of research in this field, as well as the wide differences among definitions of the observation unit "concept" [52] itself, all require a discussion of the essential peculiarities.

Important applications in medicine requiring classification of concepts are: investigating the mortality of newborns; planning and comparing methods for the control of epidemics; developing therapy for and judging the effects of treatment of malignant tumors.

The model consists of attributes and corresponding values (**semantic concepts**), relations among the concepts of a terminology, and a classification for explicit formulation of the relations.

In the context of classification, a "concept" is usually defined as a "union of true statements" concerning an object of the domain, or as a "summary of characteristics" of an object (DIN 2330). In the sense of the preceding sections, a concept is a set of object triplets with respect to an underlying attribute system. However, because attributes and values are also concepts, this is not an independent definition. "Concepts" are ultimately based on "axioms", i.e., attributes, which cannot be defined operationally.

Because each concept is denoted and communicated by some language, there is an intimate relation between "concept" and "language". The available language determines the possible development of concepts.

A concept is a delimitable unit of knowledge and the classification of concepts is related to the ordering of knowledge. Because everyone has his individual ordering system, communication is possible only if there is agreement with respect to a certain **deep structure** (generally accepted concepts and their most important relations, Section 3.1.1), even if these agreements cannot be operationally defined to the last detail. Scientific communities, such as the medical profession, present only minor differences in these aspects. They have many goals and methods in common; this allows for (and requires) a better definition of the deep structure. Such a definition is always directed towards specific purposes: in medicine towards the diagnostic and therapeutic possibilities.

For any classification, a **lexeme** is the smallest language unit, containing information, which cannot be further analyzed by decomposing the lexeme. A lexeme may be a morpheme (skin), a word (inflammation), or a phrase (corpus luteum). The systematic ordering of all lexemes of a terminology, considering the deep structure, is the **classification**, i.e., process and product have the same name. If all the lexemes and relations pertaining to a specific application are collected together, the result is a **thesaurus**.

The smallest semantic units are **sememes** [130]. They are the building-blocks of information and correspond to an object triplet on the lowest level of the deep structure (Section 3.4.2.2).

3.4.1 Nomenclature and Terminology

A **nomenclature** is a systematic list of **names**. Examples of nomenclatures in medicine are: a nomina anatomica, a zoologic nomenclature, or the names of the infectious diseases. However, names are used for the identification of objects and not for their classification.

Difficulties arise from the coexistence of several anatomic nomenclatures [110], which are sometimes used in parallel (Basle nomina anatomica, BNA, 1895; Jena nomina anatomica, JNA, 1935; Paris nomina anatomica, PNA, 1955; Tokyo nomina anatomica, TNA, 1975).

A **term** (collectively **terminology**) points to the object and to its characteristics and may contain one or more modifiers (icterus neonatorum, carcinoma simplex, acute hemorrhagic nephritis). "Term" and "concept" are frequently used as synonyms. A systematic, multi-purpose classification requires a suitable terminology. Ideally, a terminology is a set of terms, which is isomorphic to the set of information units, and where each term reveals the most important aspects of its corresponding content. In practice, these ideal requirements are frequently not realized for several reasons:

- historic terms have been retained, even after it has become clear that they denote an erroneous interpretation (linitis plastica; "cerebral", paraphrasing "cerebrum" and "brain"),
- eponyms (e.g., three Oslers diseases), for which even the word order may be significant (Gorlin Goltz syndrome/Goltz Gorlin syndrome),
- unsatisfactory standardization implied by incomplete definition or incomplete knowledge ("trunk" with/without "neck").

Such errors are preserved by the processes of specialization, multidisciplinarity, and evolution and result both in imprecise relations and varying interpretations.

Many examples can easily be found in anatomy. Colloquial terms are used without operational definition, as is the case with "groin" or "flank". Avoidable homonyms are created by using the same term for regions as well as for specific structures ("breast", "shoulder", "knee").

New knowledge continually alters the attribute system, but lexemes are rarely altered correspondingly. This leads to misunderstandings at various levels of knowledge.

Stages in development of a standardized terminology are described in [107]:

- defining the purpose and the application area,
- selecting the terms from literature such that all the information is completely and consistently covered,
- defining the terms and their scaling,
- defining the appropriate relations.

The Current Medical Information and Terminology [54] contains about 3,500 disease terms along with their definitions with respect to etiology, symptomatology, x-ray findings, and laboratory tests. Additional efforts towards standardization are made for tumor nomenclature [163] and clinical syndromes [95].

The existence of many synonyms and quasi-synonyms, which are frequently not clearly separable, makes communication more difficult. For example, about a dozen synonyms for "arteriosclerosis" (atherosclerosis, atheromatosis, ...) are in present use. Because it is almost impossible to restrict the terminology to unique terms for diseases, we should at least agree on urgently needed definitions of **preferred terms**. In recent years, international efforts have been made along these lines by the Council for International Organizations of Medical Sciences [28,29].

A terminology presupposes diseases to be units defined independently of the patient. However, "disease" is also used as an explanation for signs and symptoms in a specific patient. This interaction of "disease units" and "disease cases" is found in every medical subfield.

The process leading to the assignment of one or more disease terms to a cluster of signs and symptoms in a specific patient is called **diagnostic process**. The reader is referred to the relevant literature for a discussion of the specific problems. The various influences on the diagnosis have been described, especially in [62]:

- physicians attempt to summarize the diversity of individual and time-dependent signs and symptoms,
- diagnostic possibilities (instrumentation, knowledge, ...),
- purpose (selection of a suitable treatment, reasons for a therapy, justification of hospital admission to the medical staff, to the insurance agency, ...),
- theory for explanation of the observations,
- classification of the disease terms.

Progress in this complex area will only be made by operational definition of the elementary events constituting a term. These elementary events comprise all phenomena perceivable by observation or by measurement.

The fact that "disease" is a **process** and not a state can be considered on the level of elementary events by introducing semantic relations. In [62] a relation between two elementary events,

$$E_1 \rightarrow E_2 ,$$

is called a **patheme** by analogy with other terms. Examples of such pathemes are taken from [62]:

Hypalbuminemia $\rightarrow$ edema

pain $\rightarrow$ muscle tension

muscle tension $\rightarrow$ pain

potassium $\wedge$ decrease of H^+-concentration $\wedge$ release of prostaglandin E $\rightarrow$ pain.

The second and third example illustrate that these relations can be used to formulate oscillation. Pathemes of higher order up to "diseases" may be constructed on the basis of pathemes of lower order. As perceived in this way, **pathogenesis** is the logical and temporal order of pathemes.

This attempt to establish a binary relation (interpreted as "leads to") between elementary events must be further worked out, before it can be used as a means for formalization. At present, neither the elementary events nor the relations are sufficiently well-defined. For example, the characteristics of the relation, such as transitivity, have to be examined and subsets have to be identified, which have special characteristics such as symmetry.

However, these definitions do not replace a standardized terminology.

This can especially well be illustrated by considering the patheme

$$\text{muscle tension} \longrightarrow \text{pain:}$$

- The concept of "muscle tension" must not be confused with the normal muscle tone or with the normal reaction when a muscle is activated.
- The dependence expressed by the relation $\longrightarrow$ is not defined with respect to its cause nor its degree of certainty. It must be made more precise, e.g., by conditional probability (see (2.1) in Section 2.2.1.1):

$$\alpha = P\,(\text{pain} \mid \text{muscle tension})\;.$$

Thus, this example illustrates that it can be interpreted not as a patheme in the sense of a relation between two defined elementary events, but as an effort to define a specific form of muscle tension, namely the form causing pain.

For further discussion of knowledge representation see Section 5.1.2.3.

The concept "diagnosis" must not be confused with the concept **syndrome**, although there are many similarities. A diagnosis should be a term for a (pathogenic or etiologic) unit, which is as far as possible operationally defined. A syndrome is a set of signs and symptoms, which (seem to) appear together "more frequently" than could be expected on the assumption of independence. Even if a relationship can be demonstrated by statistical methods, which cannot be done for many rare syndromes, this does not demonstrate any particular type of dependence (Section 3.3.1.1). Some syndromes become diagnoses by discovering the interrelations, other syndromes fall apart into several diagnoses [94].

3.4.2 Deep Structure of a Classification

The main attributes implying a classification are **dimensions** or **categories**. These are supposed to decompose the information. Additional medical requirements are the differentiation with respect to

- diagnostic and therapeutic possibilities,
- prognostic units, and
- pathogenic processes.

Decomposition of information requires consequent consideration of the hyponymy-relation. Information classes along with their relations define the **deep structure**. Because possibilities and needs of the medical specialties are different, there is a wide variety of classifications, which often hamper instead of facilitate communication.

The central position of pathology in medicine makes pathologic classifications particularly important. But in many nosological areas the relations among the criteria for description of alterations and their clinical values are unknown. Therefore, a classification preferred by a pathologist using his diagnostic criteria may not result in a structure following therapeutic and/or prognostic criteria needed by a clinician (e.g., the histologic classification [73] and the clinical classification [37,164] of tumors).

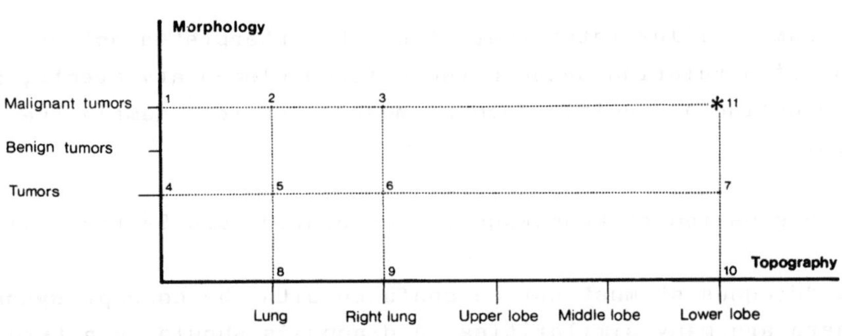

Fig. 3.10: Schema of a 2-dimensional classification of "malignant tumor in lower lobe of right lung"(*)

1-dimensional (monohierarchic) classifications are relatively simple, but are frequently insufficient for communication. The representation of 2-dimensional classifications is already very difficult. If a 2-dimensional classification of medical terms according to "topography" and "morphology" is given (Fig. 3.10), then the statement "malignant tumor in lower lobe of right lung" can be reached on different paths:

(4) → (1) → (2) → (3) → (11)	This path corresponds to a refinement of the attribute "morphology" and a subsequent refinement of the attribute "topography".
(8) → (9) → (10) → (7) → (11)	This path corresponds to a refinement of the attribute "topography" and a subsequent refinement of the attribute "morphology".
(4) → (5) → (6) → (7) → (11) (4) → (5) → (2) → (3) → (11) (8) → (9) → (6) → (7) → (11)	These paths correspond to alternating refinements of both attributes.

In general, a disease concept includes information from different dimensions, which may even depend on the patient and the duration of the disease. This allows great freedom in the definition of the attribute base and, correspondingly, of the concepts (Section 3.1.1), and the definitions used will differ among classifications. A concept should be assigned to exactly one class, except when the classes are strictly related by hyponymy-relation. Assignment to different classes can be replaced by **cross references** to the essential information not included by the primary class [32,33,183].

A typical example is WILSON's disease, which can be assigned to different classes such as "degeneration", "cirrhosis", or "pigment alteration".

3.4.2.1 Semantic Dimensions

In this section we discuss the semantic dimensions and their main divisions, which are most significant for medical classifications. The areas covered by these dimensions do not always fully correspond to the equally named medical areas (e.g., topography, morphology).

3.4.2.1.1 Topography

Most of topography is static, i.e., changes are slow compared with other dimensions, and they affect smaller subsections (e.g., the revisions of the nomina anatomica [110]). Nevertheless, we can distinguish several classification principles even in topography. Thus, the domain of anatomy can be organized into **regions** and into **systems**.

An organization into regions is:

head - neck - thorax - abdomen - pelvis - extremities.

An organization into systems is:

hematopoietic system - lymphatic system - skeletal system - skeletal muscles - respiratory system - heart and circulatory system - digestive system - urogenital system - endocrine system - nervous system and sense organs.

Regional organization is simpler and is preferred by the surgical disciplines. The systemic organization is supported by the fact that many diseases affect systems more than regions. But classification is ambiguous when applied to organs belonging to different systems (pancreas, ovary, kidney) or to no system (omentum, navel). Furthermore, systems differ with respect to their regional distribution. For example, the nervous system and the connective tissue system are found in every region of the organism.

Topography is a dimension of every multi-dimensional disease classification. Special lists have been developed for some application areas (e.g., [37]).

3.4.2.1.2 Nosology

Nosology is the theory of diseases. Its principal subdivisions are:

deformations - disturbances of metabolism - disturbances of circulation - inflammations - tumors - degenerations - injuries - dysfunctions [70].

Because diseases can be seen from many different points of view, the definition of classes becomes very difficult.

Thus, for inflammations the attributes "course" (acute - chronic), "spread" (local - diffuse), and "specificity" (specific - unspecific) are orthogonal (Section 3.1.1). Ulcers may be assigned to disturbances of metabolism or circulation, or to inflammations depending on the point of view.

Not every medical concept can be assigned to one of the above-listed subfields (e.g., regeneration, dysergic disturbances, psychologic diseases, infectious diseases).

3.4.2.1.3 Morphology

Morphology [32,33,183] describes visible structures and alterations. It contains the subfields of normal and pathologic anatomy. There are many overlaps with nosology. Morphology is subdivided [33] into:

general nonspecific morphology - traumatic abnormality - developmental malformation and abnormal product of conception - mechanical abnormality (calculus, foreign body, displacement, deformity, hernia, dilatation, aneurysm, . . .) - inflammation and fibrosis - degeneration, necrosis, deposition, dystrophy, and atrophy - chromosomal and cytologic alterations - growth and maturation alterations - neoplasms.

3.4.2.1.4 Etiology

Etiology is the science dealing with the causes of pathologic alterations. Typical subdivisions are:

- animate external factors (bacteria, rickettsia, viruses, fungi, parasites, insects, animals),
- inanimate external factors (radiation, temperature, electric current, mechanical effects, chemicals),
- internal factors (disposition, constitution, race, heredity, age).

3.4.2.1.5 Function/Dysfunction

This dimension is used in [32,33,183]. It corresponds to physiology/pathophysiology. In [33] it is essentially subdivided according to topography:

general body function and dysfunction - function and functional units of metabolism and the endocrine system - function and abnormal function associated with reproduction - function and functional units of the immune system - function and abnormal function of the hematopoietic system - function and abnormal function of the digestive and urinary tracts - function and abnormal function of the cardiovascular and respiratory systems - function and abnormal function of the nervous and musculoskeletal systems - function and abnormal function of the psyche and the sexual state - function and abnormal function of the eye, ear, and throat - environmental and forensic circumstances surrounding injury or death.

3.4.2.1.6 Modification

Modification is semantically inhomogeneous and is variously applied in different classifications. Typical modifications are:

- position (above, below, behind, in front of, left, right, ...),
- time (acute, chronic, new, post...state, ...),
- sex (female, male),
- measures (weight, height, length, volume, ...),
- behavior (infiltrating, penetrating, metastasizing, progressing, ...),
- certainty (suspected, clinically defined, demonstrated by x-ray examination, ...).

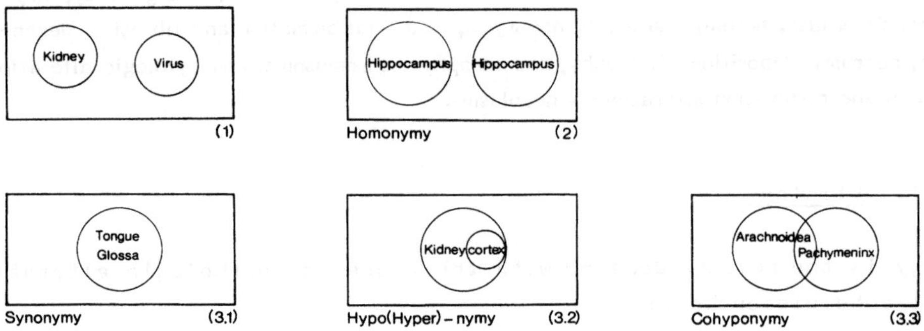

Fig. 3.11: VENN diagrams of different relations among lexemes

3.4.2.1.7 Procedures

This dimension does not describe aspects of the patients state or the conditions that produce any state, but rather the medical **activities** affecting a state. Procedures are subdivided in the Standard Nomenclature of Diseases and Operations [160] or in the dimension "procedures" of SNOMED [33]. The latter one provides:

general medical and administrative procedures - operations and anesthesia procedures - laboratory procedures - hematopoietic, oncologic, immunologic, and dermatologic procedures - digestive and urinary tract procedures - cardiovascular and respiratory system procedures - neuromusculoskeletal system and special sense organ procedures - procedures related to the psyche, sex, and reproduction - radiography, radiation therapy, nuclear medicine, and ultrasonic procedures - nursing, home care, and disability evaluation procedures.

In addition, the World Health Organization (WHO) supports an effort to systematize procedures. This effort has produced a catalog, which was adopted in the 9th revision of the ICD [23] and was published as a supplement.

3.4.2.2 Relations

The hierarchy of attributes defined in the deep structure corresponds to a hierarchy of object triplets of a concept (Section 3.1.1, 5.1). The relations among concepts are complicated by the fact that concepts may correspond to sets of object triplets located in different positions of the deep structure. It is convenient to represent relations among concepts or their corresponding lexemes by means of set theory (Section 3.1). Depending on the interpretation rules and thus also on the domain of the language, the following combinations of lexemes and information sets (sets of sememes or object triplets) are possible (Fig. 3.11):

(1) Intersection among the information sets of different lexemes is empty.

(2) The same lexeme belongs to different information sets: **Homonymy** (hippocampus: name of a genus or part of the brain).

(3) Intersection among the information sets of different lexemes is not empty: **Homoionymy**.

(3.1) Information of different lexemes is identical: **Synonymy**.

(3.2) Information set of one lexeme is a subset of the information set of another lexeme: **Hyponymy/Hypernymy** (refinement).

This situation leads to the hierarchy previously mentioned. A **partitive hierarchic** relation exists if one lexeme denotes a concept, which is part of another concept (Fig. 3.12). A **generic hierarchic** relation exists if one concept is a specialization of another concept (Fig. 3.13).

(3.3) Information sets are partially overlapping: **Cohyponymy** (arachnoidea/pachymeninx with the common information "meninges").

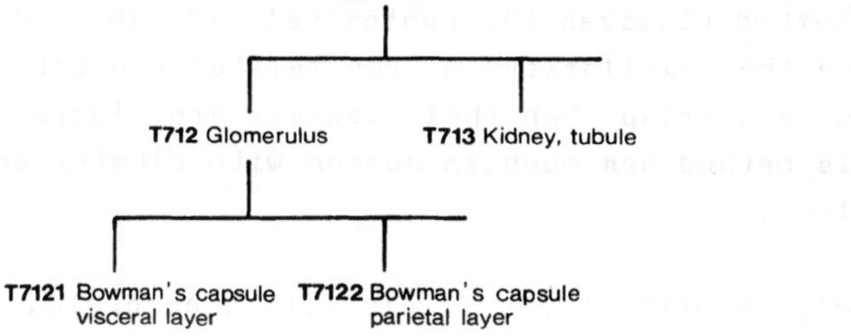

Fig. 3.12: Partitive hierarchic relations. Excerpt from SNOMED [33]

The deep structure of any classification essentially considers the hyponymy-relation. Thus, cohyponymy always applies to classes related by hyponymy to the same class. Every other important relation must be considered by lexical means (synonymy-relation by assignment to the same class, cohyponymy-relation by cross references) or by the data structure (Sections 4.5, 5.1.3.7.2).

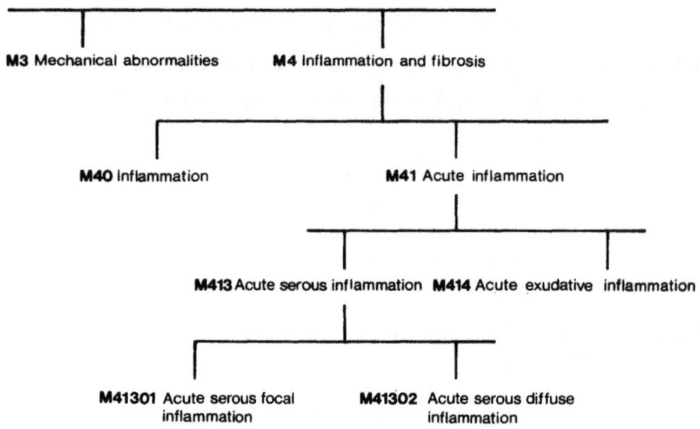

Fig. 3.13: Generic hierarchic relations. Excerpt from SNOMED [33]

The above-described "general" relations are complemented by medical relations, the most important of which exist among semantic dimensions (Section 4.4).

3.4.3 Methods

The methods of classification, often used in combination, are distinguished according as they (1) begin with a predefined deep structure (component analysis), (2) develop the deep structure from a set of concepts (scaling), or (3) start from the relations ("statistical" method).

The **statistical** method utilizes the contextual distribution of two lexemes to determine the "similarity" of the related concepts. Two concepts are assumed to overlap when their lexemes are always used in the same context. This method has much in common with cluster analysis including its problems.

For **component analysis** each lexeme is classified according to:

- a set of object triplets determining the position with respect to the deep structure (e.g., hyponymy-relation),
- a special identifier denoting the individual concept,
- rules for the condition, under which the lexeme may be combined with other lexemes.

Scaling differs from component analysis "only" by the fact that the criteria for positioning a lexeme are not explicitly stated.

If the deep structure is completely defined and if all object triplets are known, then classification is a straightforward procedure. It results in **monothetic** classes characterized by identical sets of object triplets for each element. But, because the deep structure is usually defined only as a rough framework, monothetic classes are often too inhomogeneous with respect to attributes not considered in the deep structure. The discussion will be carried on in Section 4.4.

3.4.4 Coding Semantic Relations

To simplify the use of classes containing concepts, lexemes are usually coded (Section 2.2.2). In theory, the character set from which the picture set is constructed is arbitrary; but for technical reasons natural numbers are preferred, because they naturally exhibit hyponymy-relations, i.e., the deep structure of a 1-dimensional classification:

> If a classification consequently involves hyponymy-relations, then the structure of the classes may be represented as a tree (Fig. 3.12, 3.13). Each class is broken down into disjoint subsets on the next level below. This procedure is repeated until 1-element classes are reached. Levels are assigned to positions of the code, for example, from left to right; at the same level classes are numbered consecutively (Fig. 3.14).

The most significant example of this type of coding is the **universal decimal classification** used in bibliography. Decimal numbers themselves are an especially simple example of this coding scheme. If there are more than 10 classes on a level, then the character set may be supplemented by other characters.

This type of coding can also be applied to multi-dimensional classifications. Each dimension is separately coded, and the code is complemented

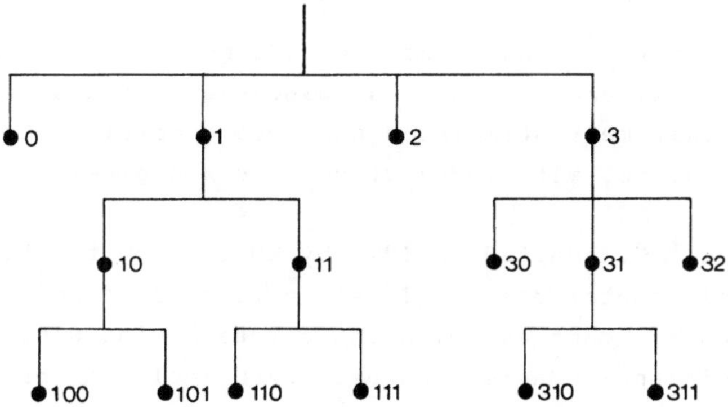

Fig. 3.14: Mapping of a hierarchic classification into a numeric code

by a special character indicating the dimension (Fig. 3.12, 3.13, Table 3.6) or each dimension is assigned a set of positions (Table 3.6). If a lexeme denotes a concept belonging to different classes, then it is usually assigned to a single class and the other information is "added" by cross references.

The synonymy-relation is encoded by assigning the same code to each synonym.

3.4.5 Common Classifications

3.4.5.1 International Classification of Diseases (ICD)

The first steps towards a classification of diseases were taken by SAUVAGE ("Nosologia Methodica") and LINNÉ("Genera Morborum") in the 18th century. Their system was followed by the "Synopsis Nosologiae Methodicae" published by CULLEN, 1785. A useful classification for statistical purposes was presented to the International Statistical Congress in Paris by FARR, 1855, and was adopted by the Congress. Since then it has been modified several times, but its basic structure was retained in some classifications.

Further developments included the International Statistical Institute, which adopted a systematic listing of causes of death in 1893. It became the basis of health statistics in several countries. Since 1900 a decennial revision of this listing was undertaken. The 4th and 5th revisions were published by the International Statistical Institute with League of Nations support. Beginning with the 6th revision, WHO took over the project in 1946 and added diseases and injuries.

From its origin, ICD is a 1-dimensional classification, the obligatory part of which is coded by 3-digit numbers. Its structural basis does not rest on a single semantic dimension, but varies between topography and nosology (Table 3.6).

During the fifties the demand arose to code not only causes of death for official statistical reports but also **diseases**. The inadequacy of ICD to meet this requirement stimulated numerous special revisions and more detailed subdivisions, with codes of up to six digits.

The 9th revision [23], adopted in 1976 by WHO, attempted to satisfy the needs by special adaptations. A classification for oncology was developed [ICD-O,73], which is identical with the corresponding sections M8/M9 of SNOMED [33]. Additional adaptations have been included for oral and dental medicine and for ophthalmology.

ICD-O [73] comprises the dimensions morphology (4 digits) and degree of malignancy ("character") of a tumor (1 digit). A code for the histologic differentiation may be added (1 digit).

3.4.5.2 Klinischer Diagnosenschlüssel (KDS)

KDS is a 2-dimensional classification [69]. Its development goes back to a suggestion by the Deutsche Gesellschaft für Medizinische Dokumentation, Informatik und Statistik, because earlier available classifications, like ICD, did not meet the requirements of detailed documentation of diagnoses that had become necessary as a part of the Allgemeiner Krankenblattkopf (Section 5.1.3.2).

KDS consists of the dimensions topography (2 digits), nosology (2 digits), and modification (1 digit) (Table 3.6). Because a few cases required more than one code for a topographic class, there are only 94 different topographic classes.

In order to be compatible with ICD (KDS contains references to the corresponding ICD codes), each concept has to be coded by exactly one code. This restriction requires a convention relative to the coding procedure. Thus, the smaller code is to be used if there are several options (tracheobronchitis). The information related to the other classes is lost ("tracheobronchitis" and "tracheitis" get the same code, losing the information "bronchitis"). Therefore, KDS leads to a selection (Section 2.2.4).

3.4.5.3 Systematized Nomenclature of Pathology (SNOP)

SNOP [32,183] is a "nomenclature" developed for the needs of pathology and contains essential elements of a classification. It consists of four dimensions: topography (T), morphology (M), etiology (E), and function (F). Each dimension is coded by a literal and a 4-digit code. This structure is based on a model of a **medical information** (Section 5.1.3.7.2) in pathology:

> In a **topographic** location **morphologic** alterations caused by an **etiologic** agent and combined with a **dysfunction**.

SNOP contains a certain set of clinical diagnoses. The code for a medical utterance consists of one or more "TMEF-statements". The explicit structure and the ability to code utterances on different levels of detail are the main advantages of SNOP.

The structure introduced by SNOP was so widely accepted that subsequent classifications have been based on it, especially in oncology [73,118] and in the total medical area (Section 3.4.5.4).

3.4.5.4 Systematized Nomenclature of Medicine (SNOMED)

SNOMED [33] follows the principles of SNOP (Table 3.6). It is the most voluminous "nomenclature" in medicine and contains about 45,000 lexemes.

It differs most significantly from SNOP in:

- higher degree of differentiation, sometimes requiring a 5-digit code in a single dimension,
- addition of the dimensions "procedures" (Section 3.4.2.1.7) and "diseases". These two dimensions became necessary for clinical application. The dimension "diseases" contains a classification for the lexemes of those complex medical concepts, which cannot be assigned to a single class in the other dimensions.

In spite of its size, which practically makes manual encoding impossible, and classification problems related to the size, SNOMED offers very helpful means for the development of information processing in medicine. It is, like SNOP, based on an explicit structure of utterances, which can be used as the basis of a metalanguage (Section 4.5). This structure may be retained even if specific adaptations are made (Section 5.1.3.7.2).

SNOMED can also be used as the basis for microglossaries in special application areas. This is especially important, because a large part of its now about 2,000 users needs SNOMED only in special disciplines. For example, a microglossary for surgical pathology has recently been made available.

3.4.5.5 TNM-Classification

The TNM-classification [37,164] is a clinical classification of malignant tumors. The world-wide struggle against cancer is supported by national and international institutions at enormous expense. It demands a classification ensuring international compatibility of therapies and therapy-effects. Cancer therapy is such a serious and dangerous intervention that the possibility of introducing "fads" in therapy by badly planned studies or by comparing inhomogenous populations should be decreased as much as possible.

Lexeme	ICD	KDS	SNOMED			
BRONCHIAL CARCINOMA	1622	50513	T26000	M80103	-	-
TOBACCO	-	-	-	-	E6927	-
PAROXYSMAL NOCTURNAL DYSPNEA	7860	27813	-	-	-	F75070
LIVER METASTASES	1977	66547	T56000	M80106	-	-

Classification	Code	Lexeme
ICD	162.	Malignant neoplasms of trachea, bronchus, and lung
	1622	. . . Main bronchus
	197.	Metastatic malignant neoplasms of respiratory and intestinal organs
	1977	. . . Liver
	7860	Dyspnea and respiratory abnormalities
KDS	27. . .	Respiratory organs, upper part
	50. . .	Bronchus
	66. . .	Liver
	. .51.	Malignant neoplasms
	. .54.	Metastatic malignant neoplasms
	. .81.	Other diseases
SNOMED	T2. . . .	Respiratory system in general
	T26. . .	Bronchus
	T5. . . .	Digestive system in general
	T56. . .	Liver
	M8. . . .	Neoplasms
	M80103	Primary carcinomas
	M80106	Metastatic carcinomas
	E6. . .	Chemicals
	E692.	Miscellaneous plants and plant products
	F7. . .	Cardiovascular and respiratory systems
	F75. .	Respiratory system
	F750.	General respiratory functions

Table 3.6: Coding of several concepts in ICD [23], KDS [69], and SNOMED [33] and their respective classification

The TNM-classification resulted from the common observation that the prognosis of a malignant tumor depends on the localization and spread of the tumor. The earlier schemes of tumor staging were found to be insufficient and should be replaced by the TNM-classification.

The TNM-classification has three dimensions: tumor size (T), involvement of regional lymph nodes (N), and metastatic tumors (M).

The objectives of the TNM-classification are (1) the support of physicians in therapy planning, prognosis, and therapy evaluation, and (2) enhancement of information exchange among therapy centers for research.

The general rules for application of the classification establish certain standards to ensure compatibility of data. Thus, "regional" lymph nodes are defined as well as minimal diagnostic criteria and procedures.

Special procedures in order to get a more detailed differentiation must not change the TNM-code established with the primary diagnosis. Therefore, several codes may be used (e.g., with primary diagnosis, after finishing **all** procedures). The basis of the diagnosis can be included by adding a fourth dimension (certainty of diagnosis) [141].

3.5 Sequential Decision Strategies

Section 3.2 mentioned that decision support is included among classification problems. When data are available for an observation unit with respect to the attributes constituting the model, we can look for that population or class that "best" fits the data. However, in many practical applications the set of attributes is so redundant that the above-discussed methods cause unnecessary or even impossible expense. If the domain is not very much restricted, then medical diagnosis and history taking belong to those applications with complex interrelations among attributes. In consequence, strategies based on the observation of every attribute before making a decision are too expensive. In this context, **costs** may be measured in arbitrary units. In practical applications, costs contain components such as direct costs of observing an attribute, pain and suffering to the patient, and delay until a test result is available.

Investigation of physician behavior is very helpful in evaluating different strategies. The physician begins with the collection of some easily acquired or "cheap" data (medical history, physical examination). If the accumulated knowledge is insufficient for a diagnosis, the physician then decides from his general knowledge what to look for next, using different criteria in this decision, like expected return of information and delay of return of information. From this we see that medical decision is a **process** where after each step a decision is taken whether enough information is available to make a safe diagnosis (i.e., the risk of a false diagnosis is sufficiently small) or whether the diagnostic investigation must continue, and if so, in what direction.

To analyze this process, assume a population of possible patients having the mutually exclusive diagnoses B_i with **a priori**-probability $p_i = P(B_i)$ $(i=1,2,\dots,n)$. These diagnoses are completely differentiated by the attributes X_j $(j=1,2,\dots,k)$ (Table 3.3 in Section 3.2). Observation of attribute X_j may cost c_j (**attribute costs**). We seek a diagnostic strategy defining that observation sequence of attributes, which is **optimal** with respect to minimum expected total costs of diagnosis in a randomly drawn patient.

In the following section, an algorithm for the exact solution of the problem is presented and its most important concepts are introduced. Because practical decision problems are frequently of such a size that they cannot be solved exactly, strategies for suboptimal solutions are explained on the basis of mathematical **game theory**. Finally, a practical application with an "artificial intelligence" model is introduced. Further information can be found in [171].

3.5.1 Optimal Solution Using Dynamic Programming

Table 3.7 contains a diagnosis-symptom matrix with four diagnoses and three binary attributes. The order of the decisions is represented as a tree (Fig. 3.15). Initially, in D_1 each of the three attributes may be observed. If we start with attribute X_1, and if X_1 is present, then the diagnosis must be B_1. If X_1 is absent, then the diagnoses B_2, B_3, and B_4 are possible. For clarification, X_2 or X_3 may be observed. If in D_{112} attribute X_2 is observed next, and if X_2 is present, then the diagnosis is B_2, because X_1 is absent. If X_2 is absent, then B_3 and B_4 have to be differentiated by observing attribute X_3. Fig. 3.15 illustrates all possible strategies.

The decision tree contains three types of nodes (Fig. 3.15):

- **terminal modes** (B) where a diagnosis is made,
- **decision modes** (D) where an attribute is selected, and
- **attribute modes** (F) where an attribute is observed.

A sequential decision strategy is the prototype of a **recursive** problem:

> Each subtree with a decision node as root (**substrategy**) may be treated like the whole decision tree. A **strategy** consists of a decision concerning the attribute to be observed. After observation, either the **terminal** decision (diagnosis) is made or the next decision node is reached. The optimal strategy is a sequence of optimal substrategies.

Decision nodes and attribute nodes are hierarchically numbered (Section 3.4.4). Alternative strategies differ by the decisions made in decision nodes. Therefore, the example contains six different strategies, out of which two strategies are presented separately in Fig. 3.16.

The expected costs are recursively computed by using the following algorithm (Fig. 3.17):

B \ X	X_1	X_2	X_3
B_1	1	1	1
B_2	0	1	1
B_3	0	0	1
B_4	0	0	0

Table 3.7: Diagnosis-symptom matrix with four diagnoses B_1 to B_4 and three binary attributes X_1 to X_3

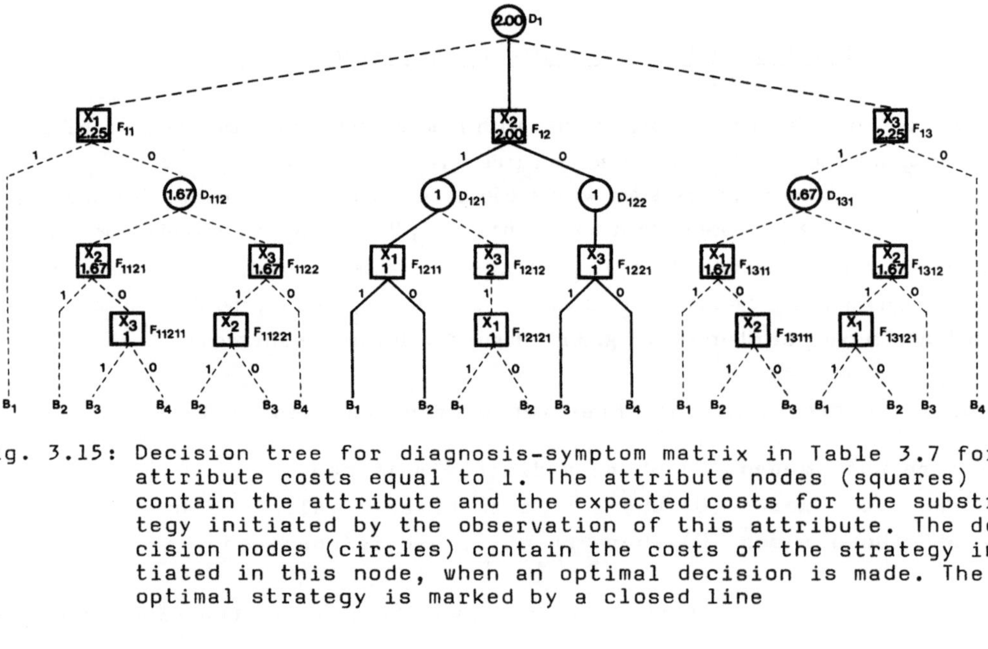

Fig. 3.15: Decision tree for diagnosis-symptom matrix in Table 3.7 for attribute costs equal to 1. The attribute nodes (squares) contain the attribute and the expected costs for the substrategy initiated by the observation of this attribute. The decision nodes (circles) contain the costs of the strategy initiated in this node, when an optimal decision is made. The optimal strategy is marked by a closed line

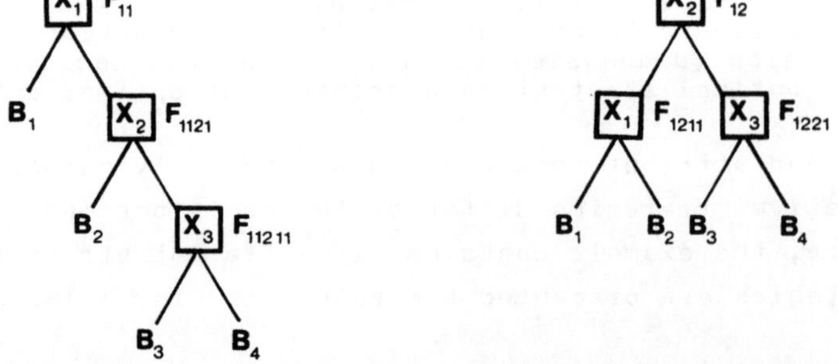

Fig. 3.16: Two out of the six strategies in Fig. 3.15

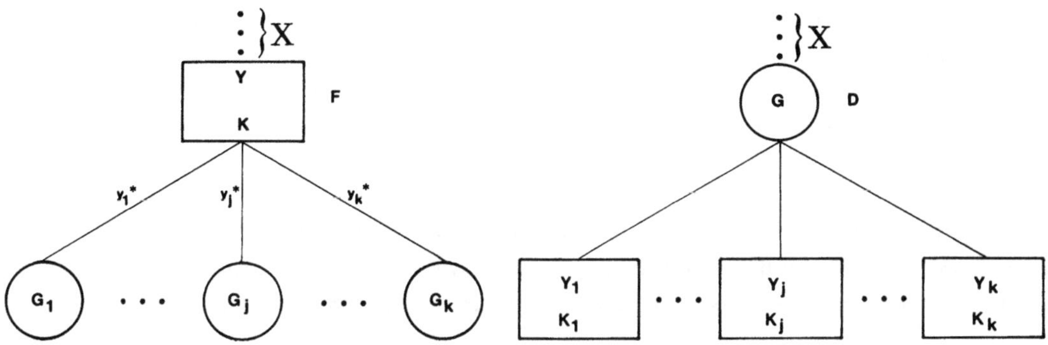

Fig. 3.17: Part of a decision tree for computing the expected costs in an attribute node (left) and in a decision node (right)

The costs in a **terminal mode** (diagnosis) are equal to 0.

Let F be an **attribute node** with the attribute Y, and $\mathbf{X}$ the attribute vector observed prior to F (Fig. 3.17). Let $\mathbf{X}$ have the realization $\mathbf{x}$. Y may have the attribute costs c_Y and the levels $y_1^*, y_2^*, \ldots, y_k^*$. When $Y=y_j^*$, the decision tree reaches a node with the expected costs G_j.

Then the expected costs K in F are equal to the sum of the attribute costs c_Y of Y and the expected costs G_j of the substrategies following the observation of Y:

$$(3.4) \qquad K = c_Y + \sum_{j=1}^{k} P(Y=y_j^* \mid \mathbf{X}=\mathbf{x}) \cdot G_j \; .$$

The expected costs in an attribute node must be strictly distinguished from the attribute costs of an attribute. The attribute costs are the costs of observing the attribute and are independent of the position in the tree, whereas the expected costs of the substrategy may heavily depend on the position of the attribute node.

Let D be a **decision node**, in which the attribute Y_j can be observed. Let K_j be the expected costs in the subsequent attribute node (Fig. 3.17). Then the attribute with the minimum expected costs as to (3.4) is selected. The expected costs G in D thus are:

$$(3.5) \qquad G = \min_j K_j \; .$$

These definitions make a recursive computation of the expected costs in each node possible, i.e., one starts from the terminal nodes and proceeds upwards until the root node of the whole tree is reached. The optimal strategy emerges if one sequentially branches in each decision node to an attribute node with expected costs equal to the costs in the decision node. Such a node may be not unique.

If the probabilities p_i in the example (Fig. 3.15) are all equal to 0.25 and if the attribute costs are equal to 1, then the optimal strategy is that one having as expected costs the minimal expected number of attribute nodes. Thus, one gets the following costs as to (3.4) and (3.5):

$$K_{1211} = 1 + P(X_1=1 \mid X_2=1) \cdot 0 + P(X_1=0 \mid X_2=1) \cdot 0=1$$
$$K_{12121} = 1 + P(X_1=1 \mid X_2=1 \cap X_3=1) \cdot 0 + P(X_1=0 \mid X_2=1 \cap X_3=1) \cdot 0 = 1$$
$$K_{1212} = 1 + P(X_3=1 \mid X_2=1) \cdot K_{12121} = 1 + 1 \cdot 1 = 2$$
$$G_{121} = \min(K_{1211}, K_{1212}) = \min(1,2) = 1 .$$

The result in this example is the entropy as expected costs of the optimal strategy (neglecting a constant factor equal to the attribute costs).

The following theorem is a special formulation of SHANNON's coding theorem and illustrates that this result may be generalized.

Let there be n diagnoses B_i, $P(B_i)=p_i=1/n$, which may be differentiated by k attributes. Let a binary relation be given decomposing a set of these diagnoses into at most two subsets ("alternative" decision). A strategy is sought decomposing the set of diagnoses such that the expected number of alternative decisions is minimized. Then the expected number K_E of alternative decisions in the optimal strategy is

$$K_E = H + \rho .$$

H=ld n is the **entropy** and ρ is the **redundancy**, which may be neglected when n increases. The maximum value of ρ is about 0.09 and it is 0 if and only if n is a power of 2.

Proof: Let ℓ_i be the number of alternative decisions ("path length") to reach the terminal decision B_i. Then the expected path length K_E is:

$$K_E = \sum_{i=1}^{n} p_i \cdot \ell_i = \frac{1}{n} \cdot \sum_{i=1}^{n} \ell_i .$$

Let $L = \max_i \ell_i$ and $\ell = \min_i \ell_i$ be the maximum and minimum of the ℓ_i.

(1) In an optimal strategy is $L \leq \ell + 1$. This proposition is proved indirectly. If $L > \ell + 1$, then the following situation obtains:

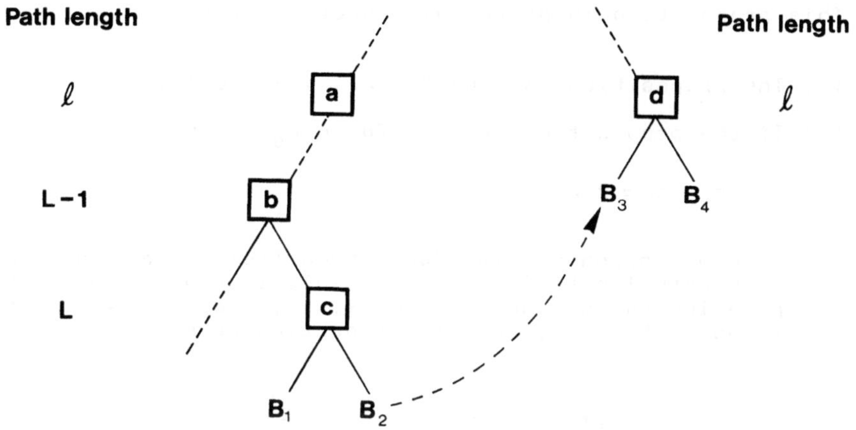

The tree is reordered such that a node with path length L is attached to a node with path length ℓ:

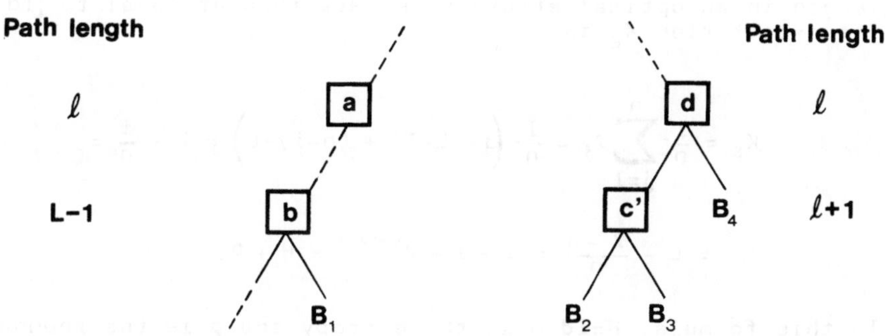

This reordering changes the sum of all path lengths by

$$\underbrace{L - (L-1)}_{B_1} + \underbrace{L - (\ell+1)}_{B_2} + \underbrace{\ell - (\ell+1)}_{B_3} = L - \ell - 1 > \ell + 1 - \ell - 1 = 0 \; .$$

Therefore, total path length decreases at least by 1, i.e., the reordering improves the strategy, in contradiction to the proposition of optimality.

(2) Select an optimal strategy. Let the path length be L-1 for i terminal nodes and L for (n-i) terminal nodes ($0 < i \leq n$). Then

$$n + i = 2^L.$$

This proposition is proved by induction over n:

(a) The proposition is true for n=1 (i=1, L=1).

(b) If the proposition is true for $n=n_0$, then

$$n_0 + i_0 = 2^L.$$

When one diagnosis is added, then from (1) a terminal node with path length (L-1) will result in two terminal nodes with path lengths L (such a node exists, because $0 < i$). This transforms i_0 to i_0-1, and from induction proposition (a) it is

$$n + i = n_0 + 1 + i_0 - 1 = n_0 + i_0 = 2^L.$$

(3) From $n + i = 2^L$ and $0 < i \leq n$ follows:

$$n < 2^L \leq 2 \cdot n, \text{ or } \mathrm{ld}\, n < L \leq \mathrm{ld}\, n + 1, \text{ or } L = \lfloor \mathrm{ld}\, n \rfloor + 1.$$

The equality is true if and only if i=n. Therefore, the path length in an optimal strategy is less than or equal to $\lfloor \mathrm{ld}\, n \rfloor + 1$. The expectation K_E is

$$K_E = \frac{1}{n} \cdot \sum_{j=1}^{n} \ell_j = \frac{1}{n} \cdot \left(i \cdot (L-1) + (n-i) \cdot L \right) = L - \frac{i}{n} =$$

$$= L - \frac{2^L - n}{n} = L + 1 - 2^{L - \mathrm{ld}\, n} = H + \rho.$$

In this formula, H=ld n is the entropy and ρ is the redundancy, and

$$\rho = x + 1 - 2^x, \quad 0 < x = L - \mathrm{ld}\, n \leq 1.$$

In the interval $(0,1]$ ρ is a non-negative number with a maximum of about 0.09 for $x \simeq 0.5288$.

Comment: An alternative decision corresponds usually to the observation of more than one attribute. Therefore, the expected path length of an optimal strategy with exactly one attribute in each attribute node is only in special cases equal to the entropy.

This method of construction produces an optimal strategy that is optimal at each decision node. Therefore, the content of this theorem may also be formulated as follows:

> The increase of **knowledge** by observing an attribute is equal to the decrease of **entropy**. An optimal decision is the selection of that attribute, which maximizes the expected increase of knowledge or which minimizes the entropy.

The above-developed algorithm belongs to the area of **dynamic programming** [59].

3.5.2 Heuristic Solutions

3.5.2.1 Known Probability Distributions

As shown in the preceding section, certain sequential decision problems can be solved by means of dynamic programming if the conditional probabilities necessary for (3.4) are known. If there are k attributes with m values each, then there are 1 decision node and k attribute nodes at the top (level 1) of the decision tree. On level 2 there are $k \cdot m$ decision nodes and $k \cdot (k-1) \cdot m$ attribute nodes. Because there are up to $k! \cdot m^{k-1}$ attribute nodes and $k! \cdot m^{k}$ terminal nodes on the lowest level, the size of decision trees increases so fast with m and k that the computation of the optimal strategy is a practical impossibility, even if modern large computer systems are employed.

Because the computing time required is determined by the number of nodes in the decision tree, it can only be decreased by cutting off certain branches. This can be done in two ways:

- The decision process is broken off in a decision node (before reaching the terminal node), i.e., a diagnosis is made although several diagnoses are still possible.
- The decision in a decision node is based on estimates of the expected costs instead of the expected costs themselves (which can only be computed by evaluating the whole tree).

Therefore, in each decision node there are two types of decisions, which have to be assigned costs:

(1) If the decision process is continued, that attribute has to be selected, which has the minimum expected (or estimated) costs.

(2) The decision process is broken off if the costs of its continuation, as to (1), exceed the costs of its break-off.

Assume that vector $\mathbf{X}$, observed prior to a decision node, has actual value $\mathbf{x}$. Let L_{ji} be the costs of diagnosis B_j if B_i is correct. Then the expected costs of diagnosis B_j are

$$(3.6) \qquad H_j(\mathbf{x}) = \sum_{i=1}^{n} L_{ji} \cdot P(B_i | \mathbf{X}=\mathbf{x}).$$

If the process is broken off in a decision node by making that diagnosis, which minimizes (3.6), then the costs in this node are:

$$(3.7) \qquad A(\mathbf{x}) = \min_j H_j(\mathbf{x}).$$

The costs of break-off in a decision node are determined by the conditional probabilities of the diagnoses and by the matrix L_{ji}.

An important special case is that the correct diagnosis has no costs and the costs of each false diagnosis are equal to 1:

$$L_{ji} = \begin{Bmatrix} 0, & i=j \\ 1, & \text{otherwise} \end{Bmatrix}.$$

Then by (3.6)

$$(3.8) \qquad H_j(\mathbf{x}) = \sum_{i \neq j} P(B_i|\mathbf{X}=\mathbf{x}) = \sum_{i=1}^{n} P(B_i|\mathbf{X}=\mathbf{x}) - P(B_j|\mathbf{X}=\mathbf{x}) = 1 - P(B_j|\mathbf{X}=\mathbf{x}) = P(\bar{B}_j|\mathbf{X}=\mathbf{x}).$$

The optimal decision is the diagnosis with maximum conditional probability (BAYES procedure).

If the process is broken off when the expected costs $G(\mathbf{x})$ of continuation exceed $A(\mathbf{x})$, then the costs in a decision node are always equal to:

$$\min\left[A(\mathbf{x}), G(\mathbf{x})\right].$$

This solution becomes identical to the optimal solution, if the process breaks off when only one diagnosis remains.

To **estimate** the costs $G(\mathbf{x})$ of continuation in a decision node on level t_0 it is assumed that the process will break off on level t ($t > t_0$). Between levels t_0 and t the attribute vector $\mathbf{Y}$ is observed. Then the costs on level t will be the costs $A(\mathbf{x},\mathbf{y})$ for break-off, by (3.7).

Now the costs $\hat{K}$ or $\hat{G}$ up to level t_0 can recursively be computed using (3.4) and (3.5). If the costs $\hat{G}(\mathbf{x})$ of continuation on level t_0 exceed the costs $A(\mathbf{x})$ for break-off on this level, then the process is broken off at level t_0; otherwise, it is continued by selecting that attribute with least costs.

Assume a decision node on level t_0 and evaluate one more level ($t = t_0+1$, see Fig. 3.18). If the process breaks off on level t, then from (3.7) the costs $\hat{G}_{1j}$ and $\hat{G}_{2j}$ are the expected costs $A_{ij} := A(\mathbf{x}, y^*_{ij})$ of the diagnosis in this node. From (3.4) the estimated costs for observation of Y_1 and Y_2 are

$$\hat{K}_1 = c_{Y_1} + \sum_{j=1}^{3} P(Y_1 = y^*_{1j} \mid \mathbf{X}=\mathbf{x}) \cdot A_{1j} \quad \text{and} \quad \hat{K}_2 = c_{Y_2} + \sum_{j=1}^{2} P(Y_2 = y^*_{2j} \mid \mathbf{X}=\mathbf{x}) \cdot A_{2j}.$$

When the process continues, and when $\hat{K}_1 < \hat{K}_2$, attribute Y_1 is selected; otherwise, attribute Y_2 is selected. If the costs $A(\mathbf{x})$ for break-off on level t_0 as to (3.7) are smaller than the costs for continuation, i.e.,

$$A(\mathbf{x}) < \min(\hat{K}_1, \hat{K}_2),$$

then the process will be broken off at level t_0; otherwise, it will be continued.

As an instructive example, we assume the special case of attribute costs equal to 1 and estimation of costs on the assumption of break-off on the next level. Then from (3.4), (3.5), and (3.8) our strategy is as follows:

Select that attribute Y, for which

$$\hat{K}_Y = \sum_j \left(P(Y=y^*_j \mid \mathbf{X}=\mathbf{x}) \cdot \min_i P(\bar{B}_i \mid \mathbf{X}=\mathbf{x} \cap Y=y^*_j) \right)$$

is minimal, i.e., for which the conditional expectation of the probability of a false diagnosis is minimal when the process breaks off on the next level. The necessary **a posteriori**-probabilities or the corresponding estimates are usually calculated using BAYES theorem.

Before concluding, two special cases of this heuristic solution shall be mentioned:

(1) The solution becomes the optimal solution, when the forecast, i.e. the level on which break-off is assumed, reaches the terminal nodes.

(2) The solution becomes the non-sequential, "classical" method based on BAYES theorem, when the break-off occurs in the first decision node (e.g., [55,172]). In this case, after non-optimized observa-

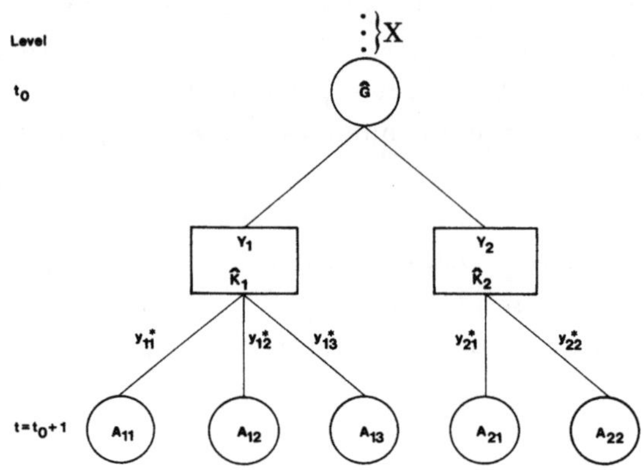

Fig. 3.18: Part of a decision tree for estimating the costs in a decision node when break-off on the next level is assumed

tion of the realization $\mathbf{x}$ of the random vector $\mathbf{X}$, that diagnosis is selected, which maximizes the conditional probability under condition $\{\mathbf{X}=\mathbf{x}\}$ (see (3.8)). BAYES theorem explicitly permits the computation of the conditional probabilities under certain conditions [85]:

$$P(B_i|\mathbf{X}=\mathbf{x}) = \frac{P(B_i)\cdot P(\mathbf{X}=\mathbf{x}|B_i)}{\sum_j P(B_j)\cdot P(\mathbf{X}=\mathbf{x}|B_j)} \qquad \text{(BAYES theorem).}$$

The relation between optimal strategy and entropy provides another strategy for the selection of the next attribute Y in the special case of identical attribute costs (Section 3.5.1). If a decision node on level (t_0+1) is interpreted as a message source generating the characters $B_1,B_2,\ldots,B_n$, then the entropy of this source is from (2.4) in Section 2.2.1.2

$$H_j = -\sum_{i=1}^{n} P(B_i|\mathbf{X}=\mathbf{x}\cap Y=y_j^*)\cdot \mathrm{ld}\, P(B_i|\mathbf{X}=\mathbf{x}\cap Y=y_j^*) \;.$$

Therefore, on level t_0 that attribute is selected, which minimizes the expected entropy on level t_0+1, i.e.,

$$\sum_j P(Y=y_j^*|\mathbf{X}=\mathbf{x})\cdot H_j$$

(see Fig. 3.17 with H_j instead of G_j).

In a similar way, one can utilize the minimax principle (Section 3.3.1.2.1) and select that attribute Y, which minimizes the maximum entropy on level t:

$$\min_{Y} \max_{j} H_j \,.$$

The special algorithms published differ primarily with respect to the following factors:

- number of levels forecast for estimating the costs of continuation,
- definition of the cost function,
- selection criteria for the next attribute to be observed,
- evaluation order of the nodes. Thus, the evaluation in the attribute node for Y_2 (Fig. 3.18) can be discontinued, if a partial sum of the costs exceeds the prior calculated costs in another node. There are algorithms reordering nodes during execution dynamically such that as few nodes as possible will have to be evaluated [153].

The above-described model can be generalized to attribute vectors in each attribute node. This generalization is of special interest, when the attribute costs consist of a relatively large fixed part and a small variable part ("simultaneous" measurement by an autoanalyzer).

The practical application of the model is handicapped by the great number of necessary conditional probabilities and the necessity of estimating these probabilities. Certain applications facilitate decisions by fast convergence and by using interactive input, which asks a human user for his estimates.

3.5.2.2 Unknown Probability Distributions

Various models for decision support have been discussed so far. They have great advantages and their achievements may be very impressive. But, with the exception of the heuristic approach (Section 3.5.2.1), they demand **completeness**, which cannot be reached in practice, when all combinations of the various possibilities have to be enumerated. On the one hand, the greater part of the background knowledge cannot explicitly be formulated. On the other hand, the "combinatorial explosion" increases rapidly beyond practical computation (Section 3.5.2.1). Therefore, aside from some special cases, these models are largely useful in increasing our theoretic understanding of the decision process and its formalization. In any case, practical application of these models to general problems and exhaustive evaluation of alternatives are mutually exclusive.

The model of **predicate logic** (Section 3.3.1.2.2) formulates background knowledge as a set of consistent logical expressions, the logical combination of which is used to select the permissible vectors from the set of diagnosis-symptom vectors. Formulation of the diagnostic process exclusively by means of logical variables is usually an abstraction to such a high degree that the models are unrealistic. Thus, many elements of the background knowledge, formulated as a ⟶ b (see the definition of pathemes in Section 3.4.1), are in reality statements with a probability smaller than 1. This leads to the **statistical model** (Section 3.3.1.2.1), which formulates background knowledge as probability distributions. But there are many applications where it is impossible to estimate the necessary probabilities with sufficient precision.

The heuristic search is an attempt to overcome these difficulties, as has been illustrated in the last section. The experience that humans can make reasonable decisions, even on the basis of incomplete or imprecise data, has initiated research on ways to simulate human reasoning. These models belong to the field of "artificial intelligence".

Unlike the models for "closed" decision problems with only a few decision possibilities and complete, precise data, artificial intelligence models support "open" decision problems with a multitude of decision possibilities, incomplete and imprecise data, and decision rules, which may be dynamically adapted to increasing knowledge. However, it must be stated that these characteristics are vaguely described. A system, which is implemented to provide decision support, must be a "closed" system, and if a probability or some kind of certainty shall be presented, then the probabilities (or their estimates) must be known to the system. Therefore, the real difference of artificial intelligence models versus the above-mentioned models is their adaptability both of the algorithms and the data structures.

There is no single agreed definition of **artificial intelligence** [109,186]. Essentially, it consists of methods for problem solving with digital computers on the basis of symbolic reasoning instead of arithmetic calculations. It can be divided into model formulation, reasoning with problem solving, and heuristic search.

Model formulation is the selection of attributes defining a domain together with their relations and the representation of corresponding knowledge (Section 3.1.1, 5.1.2.3).

Reasoning with **problem solving** consists of the development and execution of a strategy leading to decisions based on background knowledge and observed data. Decisions may be terminal decisions (e.g., diagnosis or therapy) or intermediate decisions (e.g., selection of the next attribute).

Heuristic search (Section 3.5.2) consists of the application of methods for reduction of the number of alternatives to a set of "interesting" cases, thus avoiding enumeration.

We introduce these concepts, often highly complex, using as an example a published **consultant system**. MYCIN [151] is a system, which supports the physician in the identification of micro-organisms and in the selection of a suitable therapy. Fig. 3.19 describes the organization of information in this system.

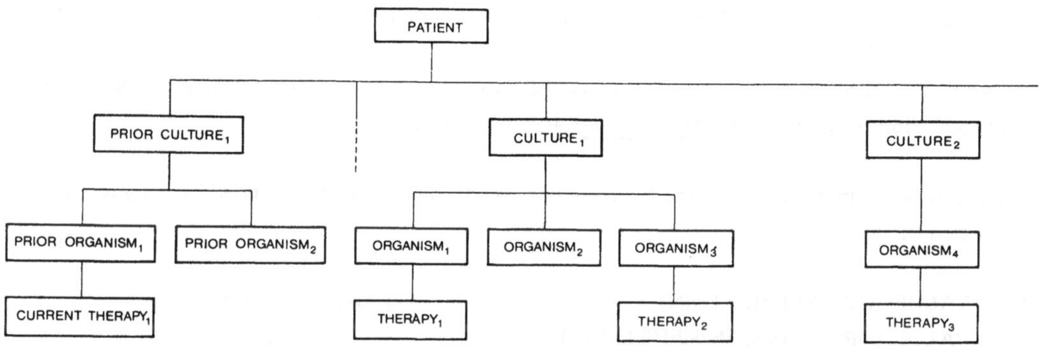

Fig. 3.19: Hierarchic relations among attributes in the identification of micro-organisms and the selection of a suitable therapy [151]

Background knowledge is formulated in predicate logic expressions ("rules") with the basic structure:

"If a_1 and/or a_2, then b_1, else b_2".

The inferences b_1 and b_2 are characterized by a degree of **certainty**. Recalling the previously mentioned problems with probabilities, a variable is used whose value is between -1 (absolutely false) and +1 (certainly true), given by expert judgement with each rule. For operations on these variables the reader is referred to [151] .

An example of a rule is:

If the stain of the organism is grampositive,

and the morphology of the organism is coccus,

and the growth configuration of the organism is in chains,

then the identity of the organism is streptococcus (0.7).

The rule contains only a single inference (the else-clause is missing). The degree of certainty 0.7 of the inference can also be formulated in qualitative language under agreed conventions

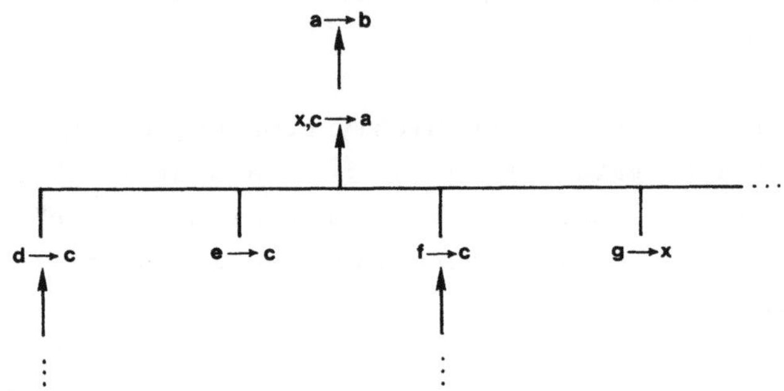

Fig. 3.20: Logical structure of deductions from background knowledge [151]

("quite sure", "probable"). As can be seen from the example, the rules contain **key words** for relating object triplets (object, attribute, value) and certainty.

The rules can be formally represented by formulation of object triplets as predicate logic functions (Section 3.3.1.2.2):

If	VALUE (ORGANISM, STAIN)	= GRAMPOSITIVE,
and	VALUE (ORGANISM, MORPHOLOGY)	= COCCUS,
and	VALUE (ORGANISM, GROWTH CONFIGURATION)	= CHAINS,
then	VALUE (ORGANISM, IDENTITY)	= STREPTOCOCCUS (0.7).

It is convenient to omit the proposition of disjoint values and permit sets of values:

VALUE (ORGANISM, IDENTITY) = STREPTOCOCCUS (0.7), STAPHYLOCOCCUS (0.2)
VALUE (PATIENT, ORGANISM) = STREPTOCOCCUS (1.0), E. COLI (1.0).

The first example points to two more or less probable possibilities, the second example points to an infection with two fully-identified micro-organisms.

Background knowledge is distinguished from knowledge concerning a patient. Patient data are recorded in a "context tree" whose structure is fixed (Fig. 3.19), but whose special content depends on the "case". Because a rule a → b can only be applied if the premise a is known, each unknown premise has first to be evaluated. Information for evaluation can be obtained from

- the context tree, containing the patient data already acquired,
- rules for deduction of new data from old, or
- the user of the system.

Deduction proceeds using predicates of previously decided propositions as premises for new propositions. These lead to the logical structure in Fig. 3.20.

The information contained in b may be needed at a certain state of the dialog between the physician and the system about a patient. This information is acquired when the rule $a \longrightarrow b$ is evaluated. In order to do this, the premise a is necessary, which one gets when the rule $c \longrightarrow a$ is evaluated. However, to get c another rule has first to be evaluated. A terminal node is reached when a rule can be evaluated by (1) deduction of the premise from the context tree, (2) by obtaining the premise from the user of the system, or (3) when the user decides that he cannot answer the question. If the premise can be evaluated, then the tree is traversed in reverse until one reaches the top rule. The strategy is basically the same as has already been described for evaluating the costs of a decision strategy (Section 3.5.1).

In this way, the decision tree varies during consultation of the system, depending on the input data. All trees start with an initial rule containing the terminal decision:

If	there is an organism which demands therapy,
and	consideration has been given to the possible existence of additional organisms requiring therapy, even though they have not actually been recovered from any current cultures,
then	compile the list of possible therapies, which based upon sensitivity data, may be effective against the organisms requiring treatment,
and	determine the best therapy recommendation from the compiled list,
otherwise	indicate that the patient does not require a therapy.

Starting from the initial rule, a reasoning network is constructed dynamically. The acquired or created data are stored in the context tree where they are used as basis for evaluating the rules and for answering the physicians queries. If a rule to be evaluated requires a special type of a node in the context tree, then such a node is created when the information is not already available. Based on background knowledge it is determined where this node is to be inserted in the decision tree.

The analogy of such **rule-based systems** to human reasoning, for example, by consultation with an expert, is clear. A terminal decision has to be made, for which information is required that can be generated from background knowledge (rules and their relations) or derived from physicians input. The path to the terminal decision is a process depending on the available knowledge and consisting of intermediate decisions, which can be uncertain. The terminal decision is made with a certainty depending on the certainty of its premises.

4. Medical Linguistics

Most data in medicine are expressed verbally, not only in patient care, but also in teaching and research.

In **patient care**, the medical record is the basis for communication and documentation. It is also an important aid in teaching and research. The objective in **teaching** is to enable a student to recognize facts and to make decisions on the basis of his knowledge of medicine. These abilities are primarily imparted by language, requiring a clear terminology. In **research**, data from medical records serve as the basis for hypotheses, the investigation and possible solution of which is documented for incorporation into basic medical science.

Therefore, methods for automated processing of language data are fundamental in medical information processing, such as evaluation of medical records and discharge summaries as well as generation and evaluation of medical reports.

Concern with the development of formal methods for processing language data may be motivated by a primary interest in the language itself or, more technically, when communication with a computer by means of natural language becomes the primary interest. This is an artificial distinction as far as methods are concerned, but it is justified by noticing that the complexity of the problems may be substantially different.

Natural language understanding is part of the field of "artificial intelligence", which has as one of its goals the simulation of human reasoning (Section 3.5.2.2). Although several projects started in the 1960's exhibited great promise, this goal has yet not be satisfactorily achieved, because the demands of consistency, explicitness, and completeness conflict with the demand of a simple model. "Understanding" a language utterance requires much more than knowledge of the language.

For example, a psychiatrist may not understand a conversation between two radiologists even in his native language, whereas he understands the conversation between two other psychiatrists in a foreign language that he knows only incompletely.

"Understanding" is based on an underlying familiarity with the domain of the conversation.

At present, it is not clear whether "knowledge" should be formulated as algorithms or as data, and whether the analysis of a language utterance intrinsically requires utilization of knowledge, or how much analysis and comprehension depend on each other. This problem limits the development of acceptable models of natural language to relatively narrow domains.

A more technical orientation in the processing of language data is required in storage and retrieval systems ("documentation" systems). Here the primary objective is the storage and retrieval of data. Such systems in medicine are frequently very complex due to the amount of data and to the needs for data integrity, security, and availability.

Natural language exchanges are required at both interfaces between human individuals and computer: queries should be formulated and answers should be given in natural language form. This dialog requires input language **analysis** and output language **synthesis**. Moreover, the linguistic principles of human reasoning could be utilized as models for deducing facts from knowledge and data inside a computer system (Fig. 4.1).

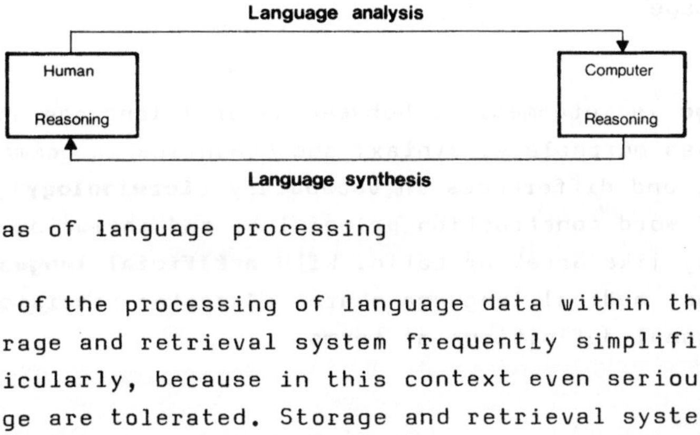

Fig. 4.1: Areas of language processing

Subordination of the processing of language data within the practical goal of a storage and retrieval system frequently simplifies the problem greatly, particularly, because in this context even serious restrictions on the language are tolerated. Storage and retrieval systems or, more generally, data base systems for language data, like medical diagnoses, have relations to both areas of interest.

The following sections are structured into **morphology**, **syntax**, and **semantics**. This structure simplifies the presentation of methods. However, it should be kept in mind that these subfields are by no means exclusive. The selection of methods is further restricted by subjective judgements as to what areas are mature enough at present or will be in the near future, to be useful in solving practical problems in medical language data processing, especially the processing of medical diagnoses.

The fourth subfield of language data processing, i.e, **pragmatics**, has been moved to section 5.1 because of the intimate relation with data structures.

The duality of data and instructions resulting from the recursivity of message processing (Section 2.2.6.1) implies that algorithms should not be distinguished according to the processing of instructions (e.g., queries in a storage and retrieval system) or data (e.g., diagnoses) with respect to language form.

In this book medical linguistics is emphasized, because processing of language data is essential in many medical applications. But it is hardly possible to present even the most important approaches in full. The interested reader is, therefore, referred to the more specific literature [19,27,42,113,137] for further information.

4.1 Medical Language

Medical language is intermediate between natural language and artificial languages. It has morphology, syntax, and semantics in common with **natural language**, and differences in vocabulary (**terminology**), frequencies of the usage of word construction principles, and inclusion of terms from other languages, like Greek or Latin. With **artificial languages**, such as formal languages, medical language shares a greater precision and a trend to more operational definitions of terms.

4.2 Morphology

Morphology deals with the construction of words from morphemes. This subfield is sometimes divided into "word construction" and "word inflection".

A **word** is understood as a character string limited by certain separation symbols including the blank character and punctuation symbols (Section 2.2.2).

A **morpheme** is the smallest language unit. It cannot be broken down into shorter character strings without destroying the information (man, nephr-, hepat-, under). A morpheme appears in different words with similar meaning or similar function.

The formal definition of words does not correspond to the assignment of semantic units. The primary meaning of a word may be:

(1) independent of the context of the word,

(1.1) equivalent to the union of the meanings of the individual morphemes (Lungencarcinom $\triangleq$ lung cancer),

(1.2) different from the union of the meanings of the individual morphemes (duodenum $\triangleq$ "twelve finger"),

(2) dependent on the context of the word (dura mater).

Idiomaticness is the increasing complexity from (1) to (2) of the message carrying an information unit. The boundaries between morphemes, compound words, multiword-phrases with fixed meaning, and free syntactic constructs are indistinct.

Morphologic analysis requires a **word model**, which can be defined in a formal language. The word model specifies the number and types of **dictionaries**. The **segmentation algorithm** is essentially determined by the word model and by the contents of the dictionaries. There are no sharp boundaries between these components and their respective functions.

4.2.1 Elements of Word Construction

Free morphemes can appear as independent words (skin). **Bound morphemes** are used only in connection with other morphemes (unclear, pyloric, venoles).

The flexibility of language, its historic development, and the influence of foreign languages produced many special cases. We list only the most important:

- The removal of a morpheme (hippo) from a compound word (hippocampus) results in a string (campus), which is used only in a few compound words. Usually, the definition of such a string (campus) as a morpheme is more convenient than the definition of a compound morpheme (hippocampus).
- The umlaut in plural forms (Väter) may be considered the result of an operation on a morpheme or the total form is defined as a morpheme.
- A morpheme may have several orthographic variants (EKG, ECG).

The following types of morphemes are distinguished in word construction:

- **Basic morphemes** are the essential carriers of the meaning of a word (distributions).
- **Word construction morphemes** characterize classes of functions and are used in different constructions (distributions).
- **Connectors** function only in word construction and are used for the connection of word parts (duodenojejunal).
- **Inflectional morphemes** characterize a syntactic value (distributions).

A word without an inflectional morpheme is a **stem.** A **compound word** consists of more than one basic morpheme.

4.2.2 Word Models

The most important principles of word construction are composition, prefixation, derivation, and inflection.

Composition (stringing together) of morphemes is the most frequently used principle of word construction and has multiple functions, like shortening by replacement of longer syntactic constructions (Oberlappenbronchus≙bronchus of the upper lobe), factorization of parts with an identical meaning (laryngotracheobronchitis), and idiomaticness (Zwölffingerdarm≙twelve finger intestine≙duodenum).

Prefixation means that a bound morpheme (**prefix**) is attached in front of a basic morpheme. Prefixes have semantic functions and functions in word construction but no syntactic function. They may be used in series and may even be repeated (Pseudopseudohypoparathyroidism).

A **derivational morpheme** is a bound morpheme following a basic morpheme (jejunal). It has a syntactic function if used at the end of a word and generally determines part of speech (-ic: adjective, -ion: noun), gender (-ion: feminin), and inflectional morphemes (-ung → ungen). Inside a compound word it determines the connector (-ung → -ungs-). Besides the syntactic function, derivational morphemes may have semantic functions (carcinoid, carcinoma, carcinosis).

Prefixes and basic morphemes are **roots**; derivational morphemes, inflectional morphemes, and connectors are **suffixes**.

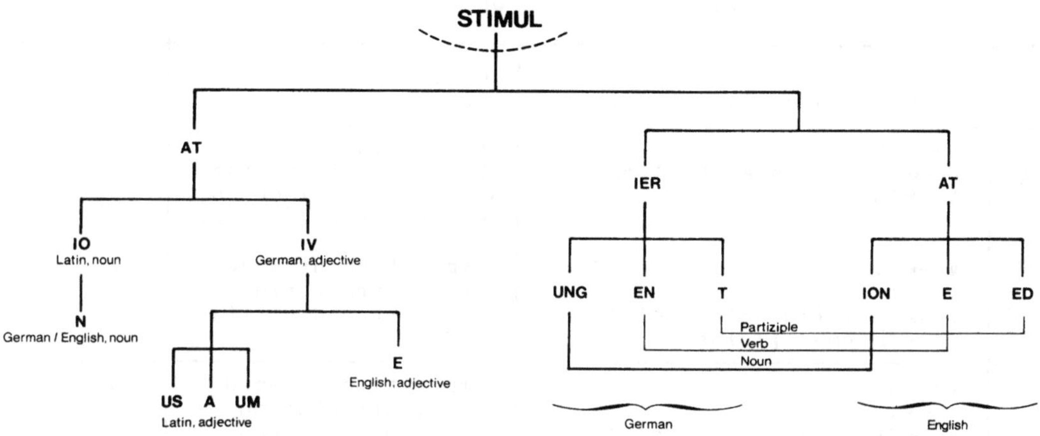

Fig. 4.2: Suffix-families following a set of basic morphemes (represented by STIMUL)

Suffixes may be arranged in hierarchically ordered families (Fig. 4.2-4.4).

When morphemes are composed, a **connector** may be put between two parts of the construction. Usually, the connector is uniquely determined by the preceding basic or derivational morpheme (corticospinal). But there are basic morphemes, which can be connected with or without connectors (laryngo-tracheo ..., laryngectomy) or with different connectors (kinderleicht, Kindesmutter, kindskopfgroß) (Fig. 4.4).

Under formal aspects, the word construction principles can be summarized as follows:

repetition: construction of a word w as a sequence of **word parts**: $w = v_1 v_2 \dots v_k \quad (k \geq 1)$.

structuring: construction of a word part v as a sequence of morphemes from disjoint classes: $v = m_1 m_2 \dots m_\ell \quad (\ell \geq 1)$.

From these techniques the most important word models for the analysis of compound words (**segmentation**) are derived.

Table 4.1 contains five word models. The terminal productions (i.e., productions with terminal symbols on their right side) are listed only when they are needed for the segmentation of the word 'granulosaepitheliomas'. In practical applications each terminal production corresponds to a dictionary. For example, model III contains a dictionary with roots and a dictionary with suffixes.

	Syntax of word model	Word model	Number of dictionaries
I	w → vv v → 'granulosa' | 'epitheliomas'	composition of word parts	1
II	w → ut u → 'granulosaepithelioma' t → 's'	structuring into stem and inflectional morpheme (deflection, lemmatization) [114,124]	2(1)
III	w → vv v → rx r → 'epi' | 'gran' | 'theli' x → ε | 'omas' | 'ulosa'	composition of word parts, structuring into root and suffix [181]	2
IV	w → vv v → rst r → 'epi' | 'gran' | 'theli' s → ε | 'oma' | 'ulos' t → ε | 'a' | 's'	composition of word parts, structuring into root, derivational morpheme, and inflectional morpheme/ connector [179]	3
V	w → v*v v* → ε | p | bsf | v*v* v → bst p → 'epi' b → 'gran' | 'theli' s → 'oma' | 'ulos' f → ε | 'a' t → ε | 's'	composition of word parts, structuring into prefix or basic morpheme, derivational morpheme, and inflectional morpheme or connector	5

Table 4.1: Word models for segmentation of medical compound words. The abbreviations are:

w = word
v = word part
u = stem
b = basic morpheme
p = prefix
r = root
x = suffix
s = derivational morpheme
t = inflectional morpheme
f = connector
ε = null morpheme

4.2.3 Dictionaries

The word model (Table 4.1) determines the number and types of the necessary dictionaries. For example, model I implies one dictionary with all word parts and model IV implies three dictionaries with roots, derivational morphemes, and inflectional morphemes.

Model II can also be used with a single dictionary, because one dictionary is the complement of the other one. If a dictionary with stems is used, then the remaining string of a word (i.e., the string following the stem) is by definition the inflectional morpheme. For disambiguation, the longest stem found in the dictionary is used. Thus, 'granulos' might be a stem and 'aepitheliomas' might be the corresponding suffix. But this solution is rejected when the longer stem 'granulosaepithelioma' is found in the dictionary.

Alternatively, a single dictionary of suffixes may be used. Then the string preceding the suffix is by definition the stem. In this approach, a word is analyzed from right to left using a reverse suffix dictionary [114,124], which is significantly smaller than a stem dictionary. The disadvantage is that this may more frequently give artificial products, when a stem ends with a string identical to the initial string of a suffix (e.g., purp|ose).

With the exception of the special cases mentioned for model II, increasing complexity of the word model is related to increasing number of dictionaries, decreasing size of dictionaries, and increasing ambiguity.

Models III to V are especially well-suited for the segmentation of medical compound words (Fig. 4.2-4.4):

- The most frequent paraphrasing by noun-adjective transformation involves the exchange of suffixes.
- Many word parts are derived from Greek or Latin word parts. They are either used in their original form or adapted to the recipient natural language. Such word parts are often translated, e.g., between German, Latin, English, or French, by exchange of suffixes.

These word models and their related dictionaries are well-suited for the morphologic analysis of an international medical language. This is a characteristic seldom found in language construction (Table 4.2).

In general, segmentation of a compound word is ambiguous. For example, on the basis of word model V, myopia can be segmented into:

my	o	p	i	a	or into	my	op	i	a	.
b_1	f_1	b_2	s_2	t_2		b_1	b_2	s_2	t_2	

These two results differ with respect to the letter 'o', which may be interpreted as a connector (as in myogen), or as the first letter of the second basic morpheme (as in myopia). In most practical applications one does not need every formally possible segmentation, but only the semantically correct segmentation. An expert in medical language "knows" that the first segmentation is semantically wrong. A semantic analysis based

Morpheme class	German	English	German/English	Sum
Roots	1,844	961	6,794	9,599
Derivational morphemes	209	316	241	766
Connectors/inflectional morphemes	23	1	26	50
Sum	2,076	1,278	7,061	10,415

Table 4.2: Size of several morpheme classes in a bilingual dictionary for the segmentation of compound words [179]

on it points to pia (part of the meninges), while the second segmentation points correctly to the sense of sight, i.e., the language user does not rely on the formal structure of words, but on the possibilities of combining individual morphemes.

A significant component of this knowledge can be integrated by a simple generalization of the word model, as demonstrated for word model V (Table 4.1).

We seek to analyze the following words: CARCINOM, CARCINOMS, CARCINOME, CARCINO (... GEN), CARCINOSE, CARCINOMATOSE, CARCINOM(... OPERATION). In order to do this, the productions for the word model V are replaced by:

$$
\left.\begin{array}{l}
w \rightarrow v^{*}\, b \\
v^{*} \rightarrow \epsilon \mid p \mid b^{*} \mid v^{*}\, v^{*} \\
b^{*} \rightarrow \text{'carcin'}\, f_1 \mid \text{'carcin'}\, s^{*}_1 \mid \ldots \\
b \rightarrow \text{'carcin'}\, s_1 \mid \text{'carcin'}\, s_2 \mid \ldots \\
s^{*}_1 \rightarrow \text{'om'}\, f_2 \mid \ldots \\
s_1 \rightarrow \text{'om'}\, t_1 \mid \ldots \\
s_2 \rightarrow \text{'omatos'}\, t_2 \mid \ldots \\
f_1 \rightarrow \text{'o'} \mid \ldots \\
f_2 \rightarrow \epsilon \mid \ldots \\
t_1 \rightarrow \epsilon \mid \text{'e'} \mid \text{'a'} \mid \text{'s'} \mid \ldots \\
t_2 \rightarrow \text{'e'} \mid \text{'us'} \mid \text{'a'} \mid \ldots
\end{array}\right\}
\;\widehat{=}\;
\left\{\begin{array}{l}
w \rightarrow v^{*}\, b \\
v^{*} \rightarrow \epsilon \mid p \mid b^{*} \mid v^{*}\, v^{*} \\
b^{*} \rightarrow \text{'carcin'}\, (f_1 \mid s^{*}_1 \mid \ldots) \\
b \rightarrow \text{'carcin'}\, (s_1 \mid s_2 \mid \ldots) \\
s^{*}_1 \rightarrow \text{'om'}\, (f_2 \mid \ldots) \\
s_1 \rightarrow \text{'om'}\, (t_1 \mid \ldots) \\
\cdot \\
\cdot \\
\cdot \\
\cdot \\
\cdot
\end{array}\right.
$$

This syntax supplies references to the permitted successors of each morpheme. If the suffixes are arranged in families, then three of the five dictionaries can be generated by an algorithm [179].

Fig. 4.3 and 4.4 contain examples of the relations among the productions of suffixes. The productions are numbered for simplification. Some of the productions contained in Fig. 4.3 are:

4 $\rightarrow$ ϵ(59 | 242) | 'y'
37 $\rightarrow$ 'ion' (88)
40 $\rightarrow$ 'it' (4)
59 $\rightarrow$ 'a' ('s' | . . .)
88 $\rightarrow$ 'al' (40) .

The suffix '-ionalitas' is generated by the production sequence 37,88,40,4,59.

Some of the productions contained in Fig. 4.4 are:

22 $\rightarrow$ 'i' (58) | ϵ (217)
58 $\rightarrow$'s' | 'd' (229 | 233 | 253 | 255)
187 $\rightarrow$ 'it' (22 | 108)
213 $\rightarrow$ 'en'
217 $\rightarrow$ 'i'
229 $\rightarrow$ ϵ(213) | 'en' .

The suffix '-itis' for inflammations is generated by the production sequence 187,22,58. The suffix '-itische', consisting of a derivational morpheme and an inflectional morpheme, is generated by the production sequence 187,108,224.

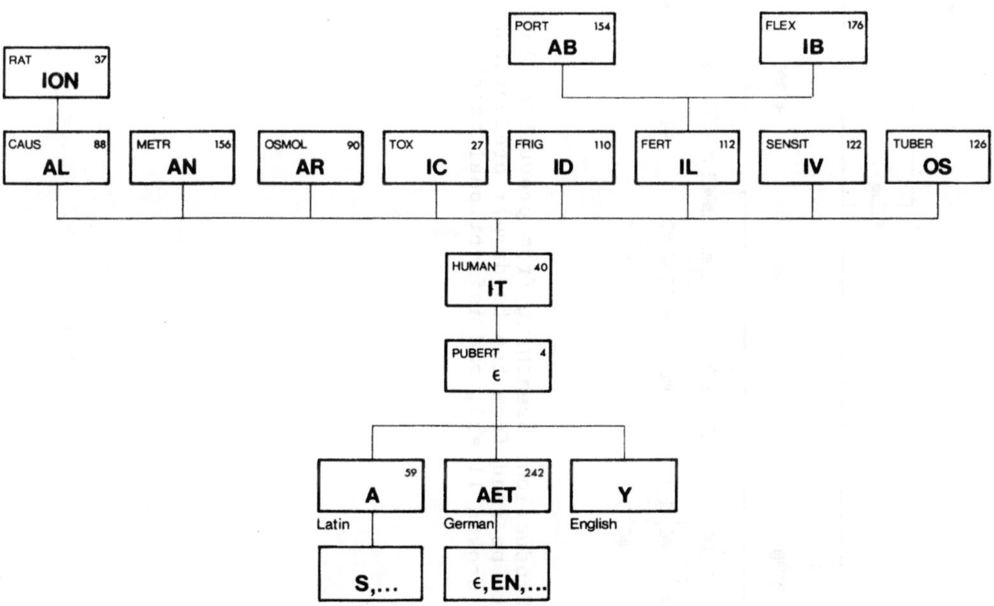

Fig. 4.3: Hierarchic relations among suffix-families (to be read from top to down). Each node corresponds to a family which can follow a set of basic morphemes (represented by a single element). The terminal nodes represent a set of inflectional morphemes (verifying direction) [179]

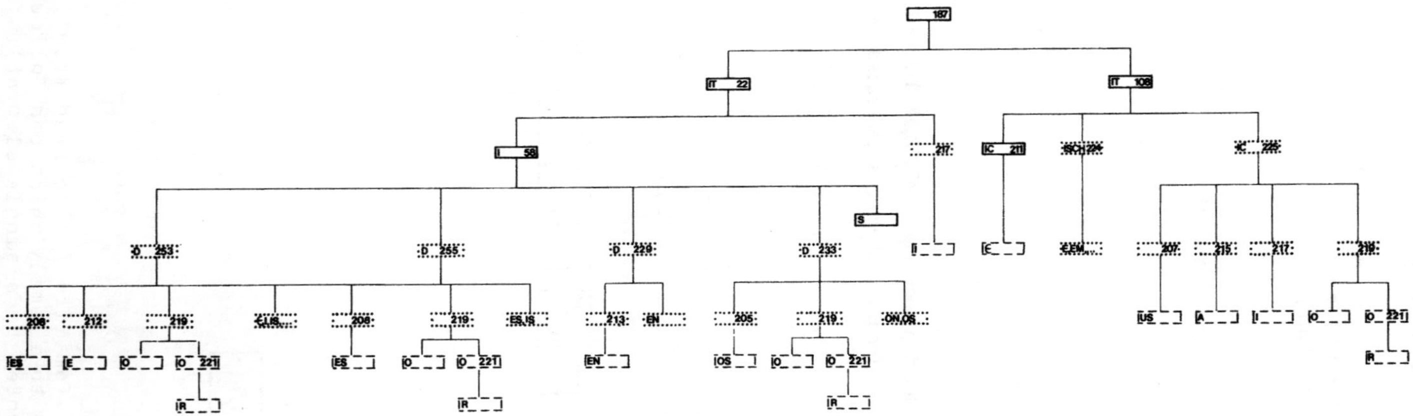

Fig. 4.4: Productions branching from production 187 (suffixes for "inflammations") (deductive direction, to be read from top to down): productions for derivational morphemes (solid lines), connectors (broken lines), and inflectional morphemes (dotted lines)

Augmentation by syntactic and semantic information simplifies the subsequent syntactic analysis. The lexical analysis needed to supply the data for syntactic analysis may even be a by-product of the morphologic analysis if the productions are completed by the corresponding data (Section 4.3.1). Important information can also be made available to the semantic analysis [114], especially, when the different meanings of homonymous suffix-families are considered (e.g., carcinoma/coeloma) (Section 4.4).

4.2.4 Algorithms

In morphologic analysis, a word can be analyzed from left to right or vice versa. Which direction is favored depends partly on the word model (for word model II the direction is determined by the dictionary). For word models III to V (Table 4.1), it is easier to analyze a word from left to right, because the leftmost morpheme of each word is always a root, whereas the rightmost morpheme can be an inflectional morpheme, a derivational morpheme (inflectional morpheme is the null morpheme), or a basic morpheme (derivational morpheme and inflectional morpheme are the null morpheme).

When a morpheme is never equal to the initial string of another morpheme (FANO condition), the analysis is simple and unambiguous. This condition is not accomplished by the morphemes of medical language (prefix 'a', prefix 'ab', basic morpheme 'able', ...).

By the principle of repetition, segmentation is a recursive procedure: If a word has been analyzed from left to right such that the remaining character string starts with a root, then this string can be analyzed like a complete word. The only difference is that the rightmost morpheme has to be an inflectional morpheme (including the null morpheme) instead of a connector.

The FANO condition can be substituted by the very effective **principle of longest match:**

> Let X be a character string starting with a morpheme from a certain class, and let α_i be morphemes belonging to this class with $X = \alpha_i Y_i$ $(i=1,2,\ldots)$. Then X is segmented into $\alpha_j Y_j$ with that α_j, which is longer than any other morpheme α_i.
>
> For example, if X = 'ablatio', then α_1 = 'a' (prefix), α_2 = 'ab' (prefix), and α_3 = 'abl'. Because α_3 is the longest morpheme, 'abl' is accepted as basic morpheme at the beginning of 'ablatio'.

If locally applied, then the principle of longest match may produce false segments (e.g., 'ableitung'). Usually, this error is recognized when the analysis proceeds to the right by arriving at a character string Y, for which no production exists. If this happens, the prior segmentation of the left part of the word has to be corrected (at least one morpheme has to be replaced by a shorter one) (**back tracking**). After this replacement the analysis proceeds again to the right.

We introduce several concepts to understand the slightly simplified algorithm below. Let w be a word representable as a sequence of morphemes μ_i (i=1,2,...,n) belonging to the classes, which are defined by the word model (Table 4.1):

$$w = \mu_1 \mu_2 \ldots \mu_n .$$

An ordering relation is defined for morphemes from the same class: When μ_i and μ_j belong to the same class, then $\mu_i < \mu_j$ if μ_i precedes μ_j in alphabetic order.

A subsequence $\mu_i \mu_{i+1}$ is a **pair** if (1) there is a production indicating that μ_i may be succeeded by μ_{i+1} or (2) μ_{i+1} is a root. A subsequence μ_i is a **word part** if μ_i is a prefix, and correspondingly $\mu_i \mu_{i+1} \mu_{i+2}$ is a word part if μ_i is a basic morpheme, μ_{i+1} is a derivational morpheme, and μ_{i+2} is an inflectional morpheme (i+2=n) or a connector (i+2 < n), and if $\mu_i \mu_{i+1}$ and $\mu_{i+1} \mu_{i+2}$ are pairs (the null morpheme is included in all suffix classes!).

A sequence $\mu_1 \mu_2 \ldots \mu_k$ is a **sequence of morphemes** if it consists of a sequence of word parts and of a remainder, which is equal to the null morpheme, a basic morpheme ($k \leq n$), a prefix ($k < n$), or a pair comprising a basic morpheme and a derivational morpheme.

Let Y' be the character string Ya generated from the character string Y by appending the letter 'a'.

With the above definitions, the following segmentation algorithm is formulated:

(1) Initialization for segmentation:
Set $Y \leftarrow w$, $i \leftarrow 0$.

(2) Initialization for the next morpheme:
Set $\sigma \leftarrow Y'$, $i \leftarrow i+1$.

(3) Selection of the next morpheme (principle of longest match):

Now let $w = \mu_1 \mu_2 \ldots \mu_{i-1} X$, with $\mu_1 \mu_2 \ldots \mu_{i-1}$ a sequence of morphemes. Then the longest morpheme μ_i is sought such that $\mu_i < \sigma$, $w = \mu_1 \mu_2 \ldots \mu_{i-1} \mu_i Y$ and $\mu_1 \mu_2 \ldots \mu_i$ a sequence of morphemes. If such a μ_i is found, then go to (4); otherwise go to (5).

(4) End-condition for successful segmentation: If $Y = \epsilon$, then w is completely segmented; otherwise go to (2).

(5) End-condition for unsuccessful segmentation: If $i=1$, then w cannot be segmented; otherwise set $i \leftarrow i-1$ and go to (6).

(6) Back tracking: If $\mu_i = \epsilon$, then go to (5); otherwise set $\sigma \leftarrow \mu_i$ and go to (3).

Table 4.3 contains the frequencies of the subsequences of two morphemes (except the null morpheme) for the words in SNOP [183]. If the predecessor is a root r, then in 24% another root r, in 47% a derivational morpheme s, in 12% a connector f (i.e., a word part $r \in f$), and in 7% an inflectional morpheme t follows (i.e., a word part $r \in t$). In addition, Table 4.3 illustrates the efficiency of word model V (Table 4.1) and its corresponding algorithm, because the frequencies of the combinations of predecessor/successor correspond exactly to this model).

Successor / Predecessor	r	s	f	t	Word end	Sum
r	4,756 24%	9,135 47%	2,404 12%	1,337 7%	1,841 9%	19,473 100%
s	748 8%		449 5%	4,159 46%	3,779 41%	9,135 100%
f	2,853 100%					2,853 100%
t					5,496 100%	5,496 100%

Table 4.3: Distribution of the combination of morphemes in 11,116 words of SNOP [183] (r = root, s = derivational morpheme, f = connector, t = inflectional morpheme)

4.3 Syntax

The purpose of syntactic analysis is to define the formal structure of language data. In automated syntactic analysis, to which the following section is restricted, the methods for syntactic analysis of formal languages present themselves (Section 2.2.6). A formal grammar is needed, which necessarily places restrictions on the complex natural language. However, several practical applications have demonstrated that formal grammars can be written with restrictions that are not too serious.

For syntactic analysis of data in medical language each terminal symbol is a word of the language and each non-terminal symbol is a **syntactic symbol** (like A for adjective).

The objective of the analysis is an ordered sequence of productions replacing the terminal symbols step by step by syntactic symbols until the starting symbol is reached. It is appropriate to distinguish a lexical analysis (replacement of terminal symbols by non-terminal symbols, i.e., **lexical symbols**) from the syntactic analysis, in which only character strings with non-terminal symbols take part in the productions of the syntax. The set of lexical symbols (i.e., syntactic symbols taken from a dictionary and not by applying syntactic rules) related to a word is the **lexical information**.

4.3.1 Lexical Analysis

In lexical analysis, words are isolated (Section 4.2), processed, and/or searched in a dictionary, and related lexical information is obtained. Type and extent of this information depend on the application and on the algorithm. In general, lexical information is ambiguous.

The usual first phase of lexical analysis, i.e., the identification of words, poses no difficulties, because words are separated by special char-

Syntactic information / Part of speech	Case	Number	Gender	Degree of comparison	Person	Tense	Mode	Voice
Noun	*	*	*					
Adjective, Participle	*	*	*	*				
Article	*	*	*					
Pronoun	*	*	*		[*]			
Verb		*			*	*	*	*

Table 4.4: Syntactic information for parts of speech. The part most essential in medical applications has been hatched

acters (blanks or punctuation marks). But there are also special cases that may be more troublesome.

For example, the use of the character '-' is ambiguous ('PAGET-carcinoma' versus 'mixed micro- and macrofollicular infiltration'). Because this problem cannot be treated with purely formal methods, the second usage of '-' should be forbidden; this restriction is not unduly serious.

The most important syntactic information is the **part of speech**. In addition to the customary parts of speech in Table 4.4, particles may have to be recognized (adverb, conjunction, preposition).

The objective of the following phase of lexical analysis is the transformation of the language data into a list of lexical informations.

If the lexical information is restricted to the part of speech, then one gets (A = adjective, N = noun, C = conjunction):

```
acute and chronic inflammation .
  A    C     A         N
```

The above-mentioned objective is achieved by various approaches, which are often combined. In any case, dictionaries containing specific knowledge supply rules, representing general facts, most efficiently.

Method (1): **Suffix-analysis**

This approach is based on the fact that suffixes frequently indicate syntactic information. To determine this information, a morphologic analysis is performed (Section 4.2). In the simplest case a right-to-left scan suffices on the basis of word model II (Table 4.1) using a reverse suffix-dictionary. The lexical information is determined by the longest suffix found in the dictionary.

Fig. 4.5 contains a part of the suffix tree for letter -L. To each suffix the possible parts of speech are attached. For example, if CORTICAL has to be analyzed, one finds -ICAL as the longest suffix in the tree. The corresponding list (A) identifies this suffix as adjective.

The example shows that the part of speech may be ambiguous, if suffixes are restricted to three characters.

If the ambiguity is caused by a few words only, then these words can

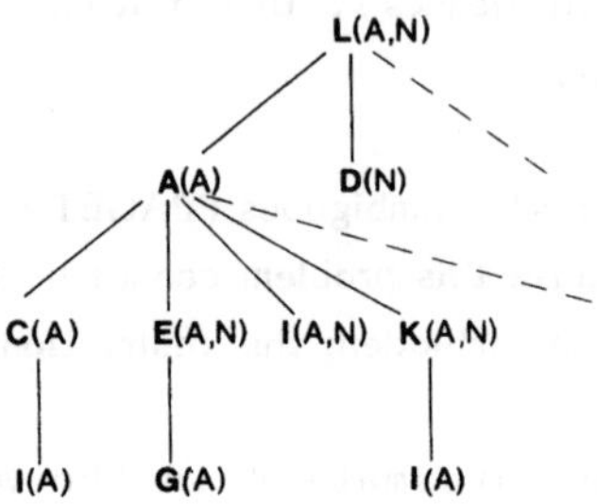

Fig. 4.5: Part of the suffix tree for letter -L. Top-to-bottom corresponds to right-to-left in a suffix. To each suffix corresponds a list with the possible parts of speech (A≙adjective, N≙noun)

be listed in a word-dictionary (see method (2)). During analysis of a word, it is first determined whether the word is contained in such a special **negative list**. If so, then the lexical information is taken from this list; otherwise, the general rule is applied (suffix-analysis) [74].

Thus, AREAL is the only German noun with suffix -EAL. If this exception is put into a negative list, then the suffix -EAL is unique for adjectives.

Lexical information can also be disambiguated by extending the suffix length in the dictionary. Carried to the extreme, this leads to a reverse word-dictionary.

Method (2): **Word-analysis**

The complete listing of every word (terminal symbols) is theoretically the easiest approach. In a dictionary every word is assigned a lexical information. The algorithm consists of a simple table search and the replacement of each word of an utterance by the appropriate lexical information.

The word-dictionary may have additional functions such as lemmatization:

Dictionary entry	Lemma	Lexical information
acute	acut	A
inflammations	inflamm	N
pial	pia	A N

Because of the size of a complete word-dictionary, this method is most often combined with a suffix-analysis (see method (1)).

Method (3): **Context-analysis**

This approach is used to disambiguate the outcome of suffix-analysis or word-analysis. The lexical information of a word is compared with the lexical information of its neighbors and every incompatible combination is deleted [21,137].

Suppose that analysis by methods (1) and (2) gives the following lexical informations:

The arteriosclerotic alterations of the media are substantial.

The	arteriosclerotic	alterations	of	the	media	are	substantial.
D	A	N	P	D	A,N	F	A,N
					X		Y

(A = adjective, D = article, F = verb, N = noun, P = preposition).

Disambiguation of X and Y is possible using the context rules:

- If a word, which may be adjective or noun, is preceded by an article and followed by a verb, then it must be a noun (D X F → D N F).
- If a word, which may be adjective or noun is preceded by a verb, then it must be an adjective (F Y → F A).

The close interrelations of the three methods and the corresponding flexibility in practical applications is a characteristic of the analysis of language data, ultimately determined by the flexibility of language.

The relation between suffix-analysis and word-analysis is based on the similarity of the methods, both operating on the same type of data; they are distinguished only by the lengths of the strings they analyze. If the strings are sufficiently long, then suffix-analysis passes over into word-analysis. Therefore, they are often combined, using a single reverse dictionary. The strings are selected by length to reduce ambiguity as far as possible.

Context analysis does not operate on the original data, but on lexical information. For completeness, it should be mentioned that context rules may be formulated, which contain terminal symbols ('are' Y → 'are' A). The formal structure of this method sometimes classifies it with syntactic analysis, but it should be distinguished, because the objective of context-analysis is to disambiguate the lexical information related to a word, whereas the objective of syntactic analysis is the analysis of utterances on the basis of these informations.

4.3.2 Syntactic Analysis

An algorithm, which can be used for syntactic analysis of language data is a **parser**. Parsing can be accomplished **top-down**, i.e., from the starting symbol to the lexical symbols by looking for a sequence of productions generating these lexical symbols (**deduction**). **Bottom-up** parsing is performed from the lexical information looking for a sequence of productions, which reduces the sequence of symbols to the starting symbol (**verification**). Both strategies can be combined. The analysis results in a **syntax tree** (**derivation tree**) with the starting symbol as root and the terminal symbols (words) as leaves. The other nodes of the tree correspond to the productions of the grammar.

Given a syntax containing the productions (Fig. 4.6):

S ⟶NP
NP⟶N |NP P NP|D NP|A N
(S = starting symbol, D = article, A = adjective, N = noun, NP = noun phrase).

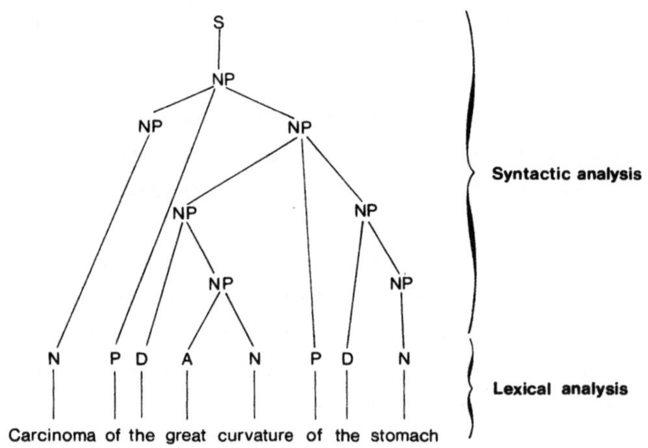

Fig. 4.6: Syntax tree for syntactic analysis

An utterance does not belong to the language and is syntactically incorrect if there exists no such sequence of productions. A grammar is **ambiguous** if there exist more than one sequence for at least one utterance.

We will refrain from discussing specific parsing-algorithms [1,13] in detail; but a few remarks may be in order concerning the important classes of **LR-parsers** (deterministic bottom-up parsers) and **LL-parsers** (deterministic top-down parsers).

Suppose that a text, being scanned from left to right, has at some state during analysis the form $\alpha\beta$, with α already analyzed and β the remaining text. If the syntax is such that the next production can be unambiguously determined on the basis of the first k syntactic symbols of β, then it is of type LL(k). The corresponding parser is a LL(k)-parser. The inverse definition holds for LR(k)-parsers.

Of special importance are LL(1)-parsers, for which in a state $\alpha A \gamma$ (A is the first syntactic symbol of the remaining text) the next production is determined by A. Algorithms are contained in [13] to decide whether a given syntax is of type LL(1). There is no method for revising an arbitrary syntax into a type LL(1) (with an identical set of phrases), but there are methods supporting such changes.

Syntactic analysis most clearly reveals the main components of a **process model**: "static" knowledge is kept in dictionaries, structure descriptions are contained in the syntax, and analysis strategies are laid down in a control strategy. The latter determines, for example, the order of productions tested in a given state whether or not they are applicable.

Syntactic analysis faces two serious problems:

- **implication**, when an utterance contains information without explicit reference (inflammation of liver and pancreas $\triangle$ inflammation of liver and inflammation of pancreas),
- **structural synonymy**, when the same utterance is formulated with different syntactic constructions (inflammation of the liver $\triangle$ liver, inflammation).

One tries to solve both problems by a transformation of the **surface structure** into a more or less abstract **deep structure** (**transformational grammars**). Among these grammars, **augmented transition networks** (**ATN**) [189] have gained a particular importance, because the model combines high flexibility, transparency, and efficiency. ATNs consist of **modes** (states) connected with **arcs** (transformations) (Fig. 4.7).

The arcs are labeled by a terminal symbol (word), a lexical information, or the name of a state. When ℓ_j is a terminal symbol, one reaches state q_{i+1} if this word is input next. When ℓ_j is a lexical information, one reaches q_{i+1} if the next input is carrying this information. When ℓ_j is the name of a state, state q_i is pushed on top of a stack and the net with root ℓ_j is evaluated. If the evaluation arrives at a terminal node, then the stack is popped up and one reaches state q_{i+1}. If the condition for the arc with ℓ_j is not accomplished, then the next arc labelled with

ℓ_k is tried. A parsing has been found, when

(1) the last input has been processed,
(2) a terminal node has been reached, and
(3) the stack is empty.

The arcs can additionally be labelled by conditions to be evaluated in order to apply a transformation. This makes it possible to use semantic information during parsing of an utterance.

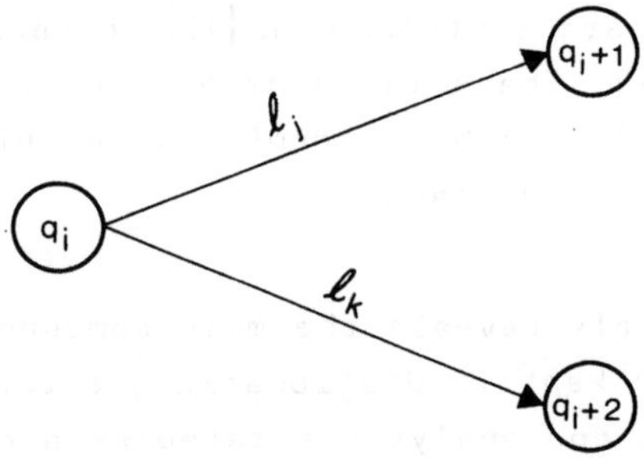

Fig. 4.7: Part of an augmented transition network (ATN)

The principle of ATN-grammars shall be explained by means of the word models introduced in Table 4.1 (Section 4.2.2). If the productions are numbered, then a dictionary entry may be formalized as follows:

Type	Morpheme	Productions
root	r	$\underbrace{i_1 i_2 \cdots}_{\ell_r}$
derivational morpheme	s	$\underbrace{j_1\ \ell_{j_1}\ j_2\ \ell_{j_2} \cdots}_{\ell_s}$
connector	f	$\underbrace{k_1 k_2 \cdots}_{\ell_f}$
inflectional morpheme	t	$\underbrace{k_1 k_2 \cdots}_{\ell_t}$

The lists ℓ consist of numbers indicating the permitted productions. E.g., the list ℓ_r contains the numbers of all suffix families, which may follow the basic morpheme r. The numbers j_m indicate the suffix families, to which the derivational morpheme s belongs. The list ℓ_{j_m} contains the numbers of all families of inflectional morphemes or connectors, which may follow the suffix s if s follows a basic morpheme as a member of the family of derivational morphemes with the number j_m. Let i_p be the number indicating that a root r may be a prefix.

With these specifications, the definitions for the segmentation algorithm in Section 4.2.4 can be reformulated as follows:

A subsequence rs is a **pair** bs, when

$$\delta_{rs} := \ell_r \cap \{j_1, j_2, \ldots\} \neq \emptyset .$$

A subsequence rst (or rsf) is a **sequence of morphemes** bst (or bsf), when

$$\delta_{rs} \neq \emptyset$$

$$\delta_{rst} := \bigcup_{j \in \delta_{rs}} (\ell_j \cap \ell_t) \neq \emptyset \quad \text{or} \quad \delta_{rsf} := \bigcup_{j \in \delta_{rs}} (\ell_j \cap \ell_f) \neq \emptyset .$$

A root r is a **prefix** p, when

$$i_p \in \ell_r$$

If we consider the fact that the null morpheme is identified by a special number and is otherwise treated like one of the several suffix types, then we have an equivalent representation of the segmentation algorithm (Section 4.2.4) in the ATN-grammar in Fig. 4.8. In order to illustrate the recursive character of this type of grammars, the representation has been selected to include the word models II and V (Table 4.1).

It is a 1-level representation of word model II, when only the upper net is used (i.e., u is a segment), or a 2-level representation of word model V, when both nets are used (i.e., u is further segmented in a sequence of morphemes). An arc may only be used, when the corresponding condition is accomplished. E.g., the arc labelled by s may only be used, when $\delta_{rs} \neq \emptyset$. The terminal nodes are designated by a slash in the node.

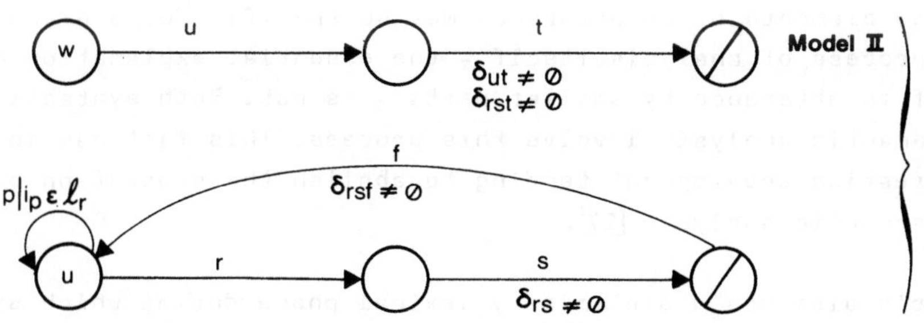

Fig. 4.8: ATN-grammar for word models II and V

4.4 Semantics

Because **understanding** is the ultimate objective of language processing, the methods, described so far, may be considered as of theoretic interest only. This view is supported by the common experience that human communication needs no formal procedures and is even possible when the utterances are incomplete or syntactically incorrect.

However, the total elimination of morphologic and syntactic analysis is at least inefficient, because there are many utterances where the formal structure serves as a basis for the organization or even determination of the content (kidney pelvis - pelvic kidney, accident due to blindness - blindness due to accident).

Semantic analysis requires two main components:

(1) A model of the real world (Section 3.1.1) and a knowledge base (non-procedural knowledge) (Section 3.4).

(2) Formal methods for the analysis of language data, consisting of a sequence of transformations mapping the utterance into elements of the model while preserving the meaning (procedural knowledge).

The syntactic analysis described in Section 4.3 may be interpreted as follows:

(1) Lexical information is assigned to the elements of an utterance (words).

(2) Then a sequence of productions is found that collects the elements of an utterance step by step into larger and larger units until the whole utterance is explained as a unit (starting symbol).

This interpretation suggests that, while the interpretation of the symbols assigned to elements of an utterance may be specific for a given analysis, the process of analysis itself - the essential explanation of larger parts of an utterance by smaller parts - is not. Both syntactic analysis and semantic analysis involve this process. This fact has initiated an interesting development tending to abolish the separation of syntactic and semantic analysis [27].

Semantic analysis also has a preliminary lexical phase during which symbols are assigned to the elements of an utterance, although these symbols represent semantic values and serve as terminal symbols for a semantic derivation structure. This correspondence suggests that syntactic and semantic analysis should be combined.

Development of suitable algorithms is still incomplete. Progress may lie in the direction of ATN-grammars (Section 4.3.2). The close relationship of these problems to the problem of knowledge representation leads us to Section 5.1.2.3. An explanation of the different standpoints and approaches would go beyond the purpose of this book. Therefore, we illustrate the principles only by a simple example.

We propose to analyze diagnoses of inflammations. In this context, we may have utterances such as:

acute focal inflammation of the kidney,
chronic disseminated nephritis,
localized cortical nephritis,
diffuse inflammation of the cortex of the kidney.

These can be analyzed on the basis of the following simplified derivation structure (Fig. 4.9):

$S \rightarrow NP_A$
$NP_A \rightarrow NP_E\ P\ NP_T \mid A_Z\ NP_A \mid A_V\ NP_A \mid M_T$ 'itis'
$NP_E \rightarrow A_Z\ NP_E \mid A_V\ N_E$
$NP_T \rightarrow D\ N_T \mid NP_T\ P \cdot NP_T$
$M_T \rightarrow$ 'nephr' $\mid A_T\ M_T$
$N_T \rightarrow$ 'kidney' $\mid$ 'cortex'
$D \rightarrow$ 'the'
$A_Z \rightarrow$ 'acute' $\mid$ 'chronic' $\mid$ ...
$A_V \rightarrow$ 'focal' $\mid$ 'localized' $\mid$ 'diffuse' $\mid$ 'disseminated' $\mid$ ...
$N_E \rightarrow$ 'inflammation'
$P \rightarrow$ 'of'
$A_T \rightarrow$ 'cortical'

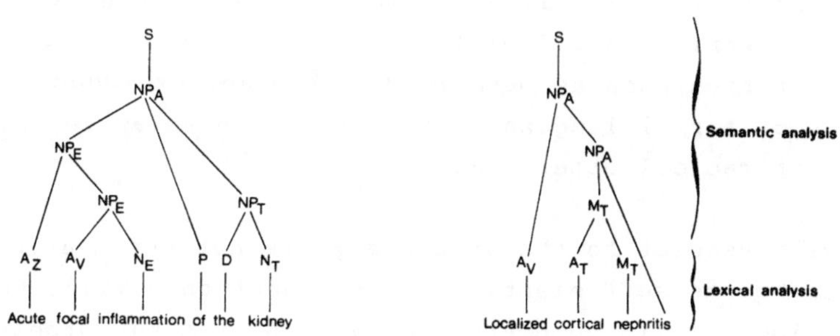

Fig. 4.9: Derivation trees for semantic analysis

This structure differs from a pure syntactic derivation in that non-terminal symbols may have semantic flags. These prevent the combination of topographic adjectives and morphologic nouns into noun phrases and immediately lead to a significant reduction in the number of formally possible parsings.

4.5 Metalanguages in Medicine

The difficulties in the analysis of medical language, discussed so far, have stimulated efforts to develop and implement formal languages for special applications and even for clinical medicine as a whole. This leads to important advantages, e.g., explicit derivation structure, unambiguity, and amenability of algorithms to computer processing, by placing restrictions on the admissable formulations. Although metalanguages are not a totally new approach, they bring an important difference in philosophy. Whereas natural language analysis aims at the development of formal methods for the analysis of existing - but restricted - languages, metalanguages start from a formal definition and aim at the introduction of an artificial language.

Whether restrictions are tolerated or not in practical applications depends on many factors: interest in subsequent computer-supported data processing in scientific work, facilitation of routine, pressure from the management, etc. In practice, restrictions are rarely stimulated by a primary interest in the general improvement of research quality potential, teaching, or patient care, although those are exactly the reasons, which have often initiated the development of formal languages.

Except in special research projects and in very limited language communities, there is a realistic chance for a formal language in medicine only if such a language comes very close to the "natural" medical language. Utterances in a formal language must be understood by physicians not knowing the restrictions. Therefore, formal languages based on a strict formal notation such as described in [63] are excluded. Nevertheless, the study of formal languages is of value in revealing problems and structures of medical utterances.

Restrictions with respect to the **vocabulary** are not very serious if the terminology has become sufficiently precise (Section 3.4.1). Furthermore, the use of dictionaries in automated analyses solves the problem of synonyms without bothering the physician.

Syntactic restrictions essentially depend on the power of the semantic analysis, which requires a model of utterances. The better this model fits the **semantic** structure of utterances, the more syntactic analysis can be replaced by semantic analysis and the fewer syntactic restrictions have to be observed. The more general this model is, the better is the chance for acceptance of a formal language based on it (Section 5.1.3.7.2).

Because the meaning of a language utterance is in general not equal to the union of the meanings of its elements, the vocabulary of a formal language consists in the extreme case of a list of admissable medical utterances. In this case, the analysis is restricted to a single table search, the result of which is "utterance found" or "utterance not found". In principle, ICD [23] introduces such a formal language. The other extreme case is a list of admissable characters on a much lower level (e.g., letters) and an analysis based only on rules. Both extremes demonstrate the duality of data and algorithms, which can both be used to represent medical knowledge. That method is optimal, which minimizes the "sum" of data and rules.

Suppose we wish to process diagnoses of inflammations as a subset A of medical utterances. The set E of inflammations consists of the following terms:

- acute inflammation,
- subacute inflammation,
- chronic inflammation,
- ...

The set T of the parts of the body contains n terms. Then the set A of utterances contains at least $3 \cdot n$ terms, because the attributes "inflammations" and "body parts" are orthogonal (Section 3.1.1). But one only needs $3+n$ terms when every utterance is broken down into the type of inflammation and the part of the body. In addition, an operator 'in' is needed corresponding to the relation between morphology and topography (Section 3.4.2.1.1, 3.4.2.1.3):

$$a = e \text{ 'in' } t, \quad a \in A, e \in E, t \in T .$$

Therefore, the model E 'in' T makes it possible to reduce the size of the dictionary significantly. This reduction may be carried further by considering another point:

When diagnoses are included describing inflammation in several parts of the body, like 'acute inflammation of liver and pancreas', then far more terms in A are needed (the order of magnitude is $3 \cdot n^n$). On the other hand, the model makes an analysis possible without additional terms, if the following rule is introduced:

$$e \text{ 'in' } t_1 \text{ 'and' } t_2 \rightarrow e \text{ 'in' } t_1 \wedge e \text{ 'in' } t_2 \quad \text{or} \quad f(e,t_1 \text{ 'and' } t_2) = f(e,t_1) \wedge f(e,t_2).$$

The relations among the classes of a classification with respect to the model are:

- explicit in the model ("semantic relations", like e 'in' t) (Section 5.1.3.7.2),
- explicit in the categorization of the nomenclature (Fig. 3.12 in Section 3.4.2.2) and easily represented in the code (Section 3.4.4),
- implicit and have to be formulated explicitly for the respective application (Section 5.1.2.3, 5.1.3.7.3).

The model corresponds to a **metalanguage** describing the structure of utterances.

The structure of a metalanguage based on SNOMED [33] may briefly be indicated.

If the semantic dimensions are coded by the symbols P, D, T, M, E, and F (Section 3.4.5.4, 5.1.3.7.2), then the following productions of the metalanguage emerge for an utterance S:

S ⟶ X0
X0 ⟶ X1 | P 'for' X1
X1 ⟶ D | X2
X2 ⟶ X3 | X3 'combined with' F
X3 ⟶ X4 | X4 'due to' E
X4 ⟶ M 'in' T.

5. Subfields of Medical Informatics

At present, there is no generally accepted systematic classification of medical informatics. This situation is partially caused by the newness of this field. The customary classification in the literature as to the affected medical subfield is not well-suited for an overview and an introduction. It does not clearly exhibit the common factors, and often produces merely a collection of instances that is impressive in its diversity, but that confuses the student. Unfortunately, the great redundancy and the mass of details in the description of solutions of minor problems frequently dominate the description of essential algorithms in published reports.

For this presentation, problems and solutions are systematized based on the logical sequence of phases in data processing. The complexity of medicine necessarily leaves such a presentation incomplete and allows for different classifications, which may be preferred from other points of view.

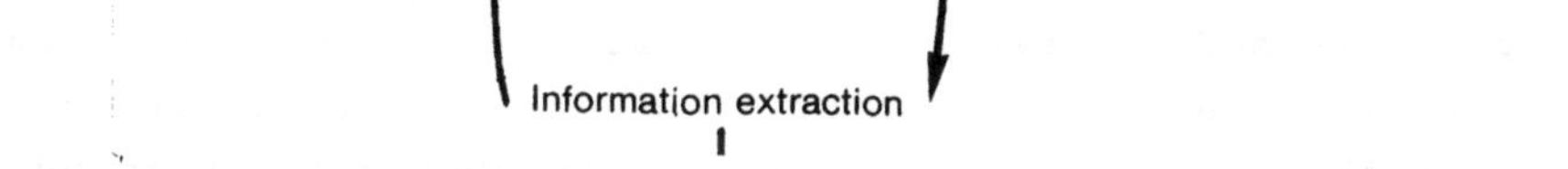

Fig. 5.1: Relations between "phases" of data processing

Human data processing (Fig. 5.1) starts with **data capture.** It is followed by **data storage** in the internal storage "brain" and possibly in external storage media, like leaflets, index cards, or protocols. From the stored data and based on general and specific knowledge, **information** is **extracted** and is also stored. In goal-oriented information processing one information may be that new data have to be acquired. The stored data are the basis for **information retrieval.**

This schema is used here to classify electronic data processing (EDP) into larger subfields. Because humans communicate with a computer system, man-machine interfaces are required. Data capture by the computer system is usually called **data input** and thus distinguished from **data capture** by humans.

Two communicating individuals have to "understand" each other. Because human encoding is normally different from machine encoding, one must learn the other's language or both must communicate in a common language.

In the development of computers as mathematical machines the importance of **language** as a means of communication has long been underestimated; but for some years now many failures have demonstrated that a language processing capability increases in importance as computer systems are integrated into routine work. Because the user of a computer system is more often not a computer specialist, the common language has to be as near as possible to the natural language. This is especially true if the individual involved in an interactive system is the patient, as in computer-supported medical history taking (Section 5.1.3.5).

At present, there are no algorithms, which process the totality of natural language in a comprehensive manner. Therefore, communication must be made through a formal language. Special scientific terminologies with their far-reaching formalization have been demonstrated to be a good basis for such a formal language, and there exist several systems that allow natural language understanding in limited domains.

Translation of language input into the internal computer language is a part of **language analysis** (Chapter 4). Translation from an internal computer language into the language for communication is called **language synthesis** (Section 5.5.1). In spite of this symmetry, the technical problems are of different degrees of complexity, because it is easier for the human to understand a message in a formal language than to formulate such a message. Therefore, the "output" language of a computer is often more formalized than the "input" language. Both subfields of language processing are completed by the application of linguistic principles to the organization of knowledge and problem solving (Fig. 4.1 in Chapter 4).

Data input is to be distinguished from **data acquisition,** which comprises all activities involved in transcribing the data to machine-readable **storage.** Data acquisition and data input are primarily determined by the type of data, the organization of data capture, and the available technical equipment.

Data input is followed by **data storage.** The deep structure of the data is formulated according to a **data model** and the logical **data structure,** so that it can be mapped onto the physical data structure for data storage.

For **information extraction** data have to be extracted from messages overlaid with noise. This phase involves data compression methods such as: extraction of parameters, integration of information, and formation of complex data for information capture at a higher semantic level.

Information has to be made available to a user and, while doing so, the amount and type of information has to be adapted to his needs. Too much data may be as harmful as too little. The methods for **information retrieval** depend on the users' needs and the available technical equipment.

These four components merge indefinitely into each other; this often makes it difficult to classify an algorithm. Depending on the problem, it is even possible that the phases are arranged in cycles.

5.1 Data Models, Data Structures

In several preceding sections, observation units, attributes, and relations have been discussed. A student may be confused by the vagueness of the nomenclatures and the overlapping of concepts. In statistics there are attributes, values, and data (Section 3.1) and in the theory of programming languages there are objects, values, and denotations (Section 2.2.6.1).

In this section we define the most important fundamental concepts and their relations to analogous concepts in statistics and other subfields of informatics. We define the concept of relation, which is well-suited for formulating knowledge, both the background knowledge represented in the **deep structure** (attribute structure) and the specific knowledge concerning an observation unit represented in object triplets (Section 3.1.1).

Data models (Section 5.1.1) and data structures (Section 5.1.2) are explained on the basis of the fundamental concepts.

The starting point is the **object triplet** for formulation of knowledge (information) about observation units and consists of an **observation unit**, an **attribute**, and a **value.** All information processing is based on this fundamental unit. Each one of the three components has to be denoted. Such denotations are names in their most general form (see "coding" in Section 2.2.2).

A name for a realization of the observation unit "patient" may be "Smith" as well as '7700123' (medical record number) or '240631124' (ID-number, Section 5.1.3.7.1).

The concept value in formal languages marks the correlation between an attribute and its value. Message and datum are essentially synonymous concepts. They designate the information as in transmission (message) or in processing (datum) (see DIN 44300). The concept of object is essentially identical with the realization of an object triplet and must be distinguished from an object in systems analysis.

Object triplets can be represented in different ways. The specific form selected in a theory would be of minor interest, except that the relationship to the operators indicates that the representation affects the possibility of formulation and, therefore, determines the class of solvable problems. In this sense, the possible representations as part of the language of a theory have an influence on reasoning similar to the influence of natural language.

A frequently used representation is the **list**, corresponding to the "function" in predicate logic (Section 3.3.1.2.2):

(observation unit,attribute,value).

One object may be (SMITH, RR_{syst}, 210) (RR_{syst} = systolic blood pressure).

Another representation is derived from graph theory:

It consists of **nodes** and **arcs**. In this representation, the attribute is usually called **relation** (Section 5.1.2.3).

The "relation" is well-known in several fields, but frequently represents different concepts (Section 5.1.1.1). In this respect, informatics is no better than medicine. A well-defined terminology is preferable, especially for students; but our purpose here is not standardization of the terminology of informatics. Because the interested reader may be even more confused by a standardized terminology in this text different from the literature, only the problems shall be mentioned.

Attributes may be interrelated. The set of all relations between attributes constitutes the **deep structure** of the real world model (Section 3.1.1).

If we observe the attributes RR_{syst} and RR_{diast} in possibly different observation units, we obtain the following object triplets:

$$\left\{\begin{array}{l}(\text{observation unit, } RR_{syst}, \text{ value}) \\ (\text{observation unit, } RR_{diast}, \text{ value})\end{array}\right\}.$$

An important relation exists if both observation units are identical.

The relevant medical relation between "RR_{syst}" and "RR_{diast}" is closer than, for example, between "RR_{syst}" and "color of eyes". This relation cannot be formalized any further, because relations are defined among realizations of observation units and values and not among attributes (in this example, the generic hierarchic relation between "RR_{syst}" or "RR_{diast}" and the attribute "blood pressure", Section 3.4.2.2).

The connection of object triplets with relations among attributes can be established if "values" may themselves be attributes (attribute "blood pressure" with values "RR_{syst}" and "RR_{diast}") (**compound** attribute, Section 3.1.1).

Formalized as an object triplet, we get

(*,blood pressure,RR_{syst}) or (*,blood pressure,RR_{diast}).

The observation unit '*' signals that the object triplet expresses a relation between attributes. Because observation units and attributes are in a dual relation, "blood pressure" can also be interpreted as an observation unit on which the attributes "RR_{syst}" and "RR_{diast}" are observed:

(blood pressure,RR_{syst},*) or (blood pressure,RR_{diast},*).

According to this duality, the recursive combination of object triplets from the deep structure with object triplets for "normal" observation units may be interpreted in two ways:

If in patient "Smith" a systolic blood pressure of 210 mm Hg is observed,

(SMITH, RR_{syst}, 210),

then by interpretation of "blood pressure" as an attribute, the compound object triplet is formed:

(SMITH, blood pressure, (RR_{syst}, 210))

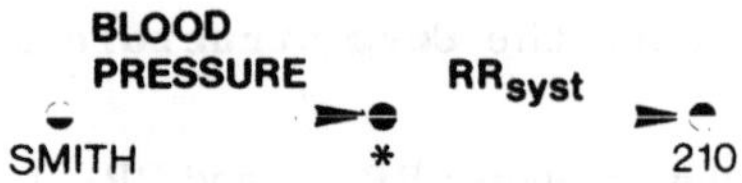

By interpretation of "blood pressure" as an observation unit, the compound object triplet is formed:

((SMITH, blood pressure), RR_{syst}, 210)

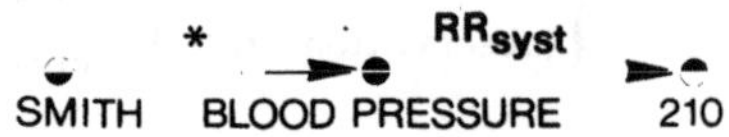

However this recursive combination is carried out, the difference between the two types of relations disappears. Both are homogeneously defined on the set of values of attributes. This fact cannot be overestimated, because object triplets may serve as a formalism for representing information and present the formal basis for knowledge representation and semantic analysis.

5.1.1 Data Models

The set of all data in the context of an application stored in a computer is the **data base**. It must be structured, because useful processing requires not only data but also relations. The structure appears as a set of related records, where each record is composed of data for associated attributes. The **data model** is the concept for structuring and formalization. Its most important part is the definition of operators, by means of which the data base is transformed from one state to another. The concrete realization of the data model by definition of the objects is the **data base schema**. It is formulated by means of a **data description language** (DDL). The **data manipulation language** (DML) contains the language for using the operators.

5.1.1.1 Relational Model

The relational model [30,31,142,173] is based on the model introduced in Table 3.3 for describing an observation unit by an attribute vector. The arrangement of these vectors in a table is a **relation** and is denoted by a name (Table 5.1).

Each column of a relation corresponds to an **attribute** and each row corresponds to an observation unit (**tuplet**) (in Table 5.1 each tuplet is a triplet).

DATE	TIME	TEMP
3.7.78	8.00	36.8
3.7.78	12.00	37.4
3.7.78	16.00	38.1
4.7.78	8.00	36.9
⋮	⋮	⋮
⋮	⋮	⋮

Table 5.1: Representation of the relation temperature

Each relation is identified by an attribute or a combination of attributes (**key**). The key represents the observation unit, i.e., two arbitrary tuplets must be different.

The **relational algebra** is principally based on set theory. It contains operators and rules for processing relations.

Special programming languages facilitate the formulation of operations on such relations (SEQUEL [11,25], ALPHA [30]).

In Section 3.2 the symmetry between the representations of observation units and attributes is pointed out. It is reflected here in the fact that the table can be interpreted as an array of structures (tuplets) as well as a structure of arrays (attributes) (Section 5.1.2.2).

5.1.1.2 Hierarchic Model

In the hierarchic model the hyponymy-relation among objects is represented with special ease.

In Table 5.1 the time associated with the datum for the temperature is recorded under the heading of the calendar date. An equivalent representation of this relation is the following structure of a primitive object (DATE) and an array of structures (left: structure, right: realization):

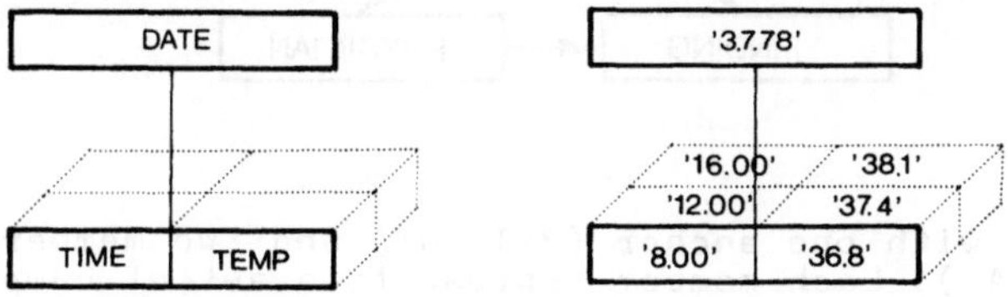

In hierarchic compound objects, substructures are **segments** and subordinated segments are **dependent** segments. As in a tree, each segment may depend on no more than one segment. The only segment depending on no other segment is called the **root** (segment). It must identify the object in a data base (among all realizations of the object there are no two realizations with the same value of the root). Therefore, the root has the function of an identifying name or **key**.

A segment may have several dependent sets of segments. To distinguish these sets, each element of a set must be a realization of the same structure. This structure must be different from the structure of the father (Section 5.1.2.2) and from the structures of the brothers (sets of segments depending on the same segment).

The concrete realization of a hierarchic model contains the definitions of the contents of the segments and of the hierarchic relations.

For example, the Information Management System (IMS) produced by the IBM Corporation is based on the hierarchic model.

5.1.1.3 Network Model

The network model extends the hierarchic model by removing the requirement that each segment can have only one father.

The data base consists of **sets**. Each set has an **anchor** and a set of **members**. Fig. 5.2 contains a simple example of a network.

The network model is further elaborated in Section 5.1.2.3.

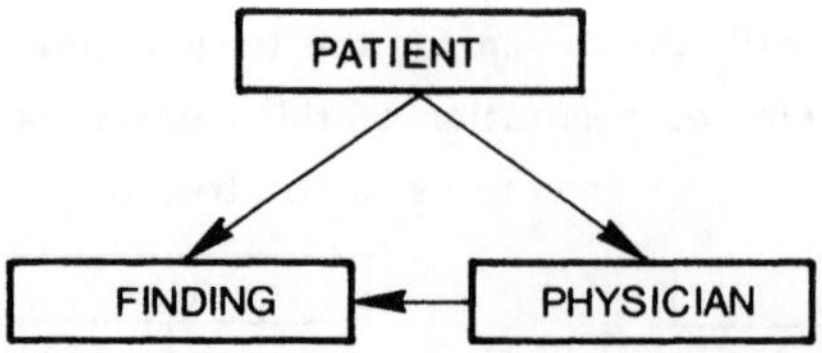

Fig. 5.2: Network with one anchor (PATIENT) and two members (FINDING, PHYSICIAN). Each member represents a set of compound objects

5.1.2 Data Structures

The (logical) data structure is a concrete arrangement of data, for which an algorithm can be formulated by establishing the relations among data and object triplets.

A realization of the data structure is an **object**. It contains the data for a realization of the observation unit (i.e., only the component value of the object triplet).

Data for inpatients are to be collected with the following primitive attributes (Fig. 5.3):

Name, hospital, calendar date, $time_1$, $time_2$, $time_3$, and at the three different times temperature and pulse rate. The following relations may be defined:

(1) The patient "name" is in "hospital".
(2) In "hospital" data are captured at times determined by "calendar date" and "time".
(3) The data for "temperature" and "pulse rate" correspond to the same time.

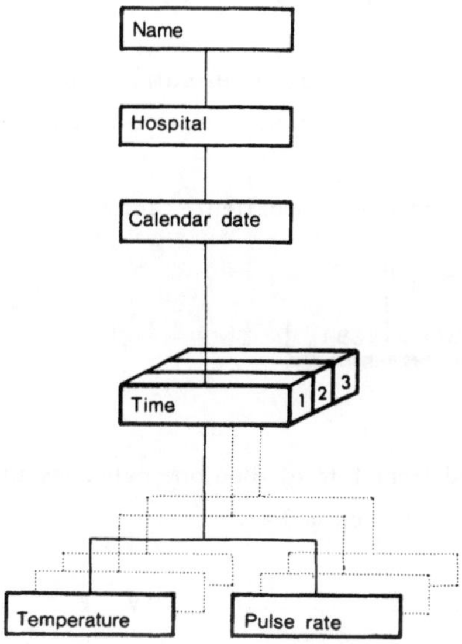

Fig. 5.3: Data structure with several attributes observed in inpatients

For a complete description of a node of the structure the name of the attribute and the position in the structure is necessary. For the description of the object it is additionally necessary to give the denotations and the interpretation rules for the data to retrieve the values (Section 2.2.6.1).

If the name of the attribute "temperature" is TEMP, the denotation of the value is "36.8", and the interpretation rule is "decimal number", then the value is "thirty six point eight".

5.1.2.1 Primitive Objects

If the data structure contains a single primitive attribute, then the corresponding objects are **primitive objects**. They are classified into **types** according to the operations (Section 2.2.6.1), which are defined on them. All objects, for which the same set of operations is defined, are of the same type. The details distinguished in informatics, which may depend on the programming language, shall not be discussed here.

5.1.2.2 Compound Objects

For many applications it is convenient to handle related attributes as compound attributes denoted by a single name. The **compound** object consists of **components**. Each component corresponds to a (compound) attribute.

In an **array** all components are of the same type. Therefore, it suffices to name the array and to specify each component by its consecutive number.

Thus, one can arrange the temperature of a patient, captured at three different times, in an array TEMP:

TEMP	36.8	37.4	38.1

If the components are numbered from 1 to n, then one retrieves the value of the third component of the array, TEMP(3), by counting as 38.1.

In a **structure** (**record**) the components may be of different type.

If the time of the capture of temperature and the captured value are to be arranged together, then the compound object is named BTEMP and the respective components are individually named (left: structure, right: realization):

BTEMP	DATE	TIME	TEMP	3.7.78	8.00	36.8

Compound objects can themselves be composed on higher levels. For example, the data according to temperature of a patient are arranged in an array of structures (Fig. 5.1).

A data structure is **self-explaining**, when the compound object contains paired primitive objects such that one primitive object is the denotation of the attribute, and the other primitive object is its value. In a self-explaining data structure, the attribute is explicitly determined and is not implicitly determined by its position in the structure. Therefore, each attribute is processed as a value of a compound attribute.

If the character strings 'PAT_NAME', 'CAL_DAT', and 'BO_TEMP1' are predefined, then the structure in Fig. 5.4 is self-explaining. Note that 'PAT_NAME' is a constant and NAME is a variable for the primitive object.

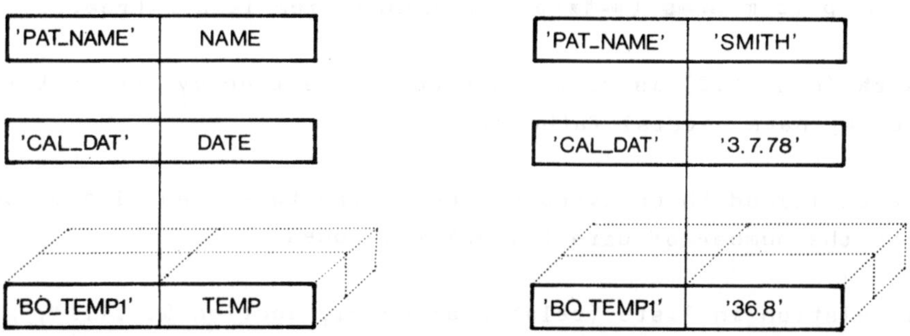

Fig. 5.4: Array of structures containing the data for the temperature of a patient (left) and realization of this structure (right)

If the components of an object triplet are individually denoted, then a data structure may be defined for the object triplet itself (Fig. 5.5).

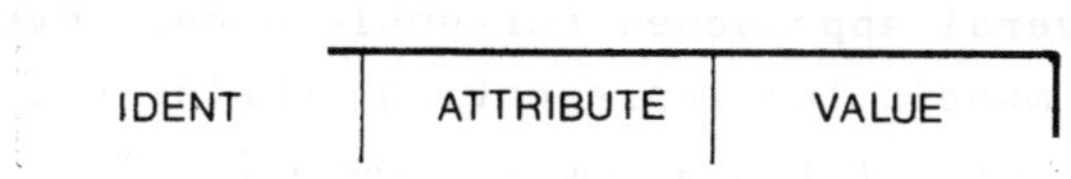

Fig. 5.5: Object triplet with the primitive attributes IDENT (identification of the observation unit), ATTRIBUTE, and VALUE

Because structures are recursively defined, i.e., components (**modes**) may themselves be structures, complex **macro-structures** can be built [82]. The most important operations on such structures are insertion, update, and deletion of nodes and searching for certain nodes depending on position and/or content. To perform these operations, the nodes must be linked.

A **list** contains only the relative position of the node as structural information. If the nodes are numbered consecutively, then a head and a tail of the list can be distinguished.

Frequently in practical applications, lists are changed at one or both ends only. Such special lists are:

stack: insertions and deletions are done at the same end ("last-in-first-out", LIFO) (blind ending siding in a rail yard),

queue: insertions are done at one end and deletions are done at the other end ("first-in-first-out", FIFO) (waiting line in front of a counter).

A **tree** consists of nodes and branches to other nodes. A detailed definition of trees is omitted here, because the structure is rather descriptive (Fig. 4.2-4.6, 4.9). Each node (except the **root**) has exactly one **father** and up to m **sons** (**m-tree**). A **binary tree** is a 2-tree.

The **network** (Fig. 5.2) is distinguished from a tree by the fact that each node may have several fathers.

The above-explained three types of macro-structures can also be characterized by the number of directly related nodes:

- 1-1-relation in lists (relational model, Section 5.1.1.1),
- 1-m-relation in trees (hierarchic model, Section 5.1.1.2),
- n-m-relation in networks (network model, Section 5.1.1.3).

5.1.2.3 Knowledge Representation

In this section, several approaches currently under investigation are presented to develop models for representing complex situations ("facts"). These models may be interpreted as memory models for the human long-term memory. Representation of knowledge, which can be represented as formulas (e.g., the formula for calculation of the arithmetic mean), is not the subject of this section.

In Section 3.3.1.2.2 the mathematical theory of predicate logic was introduced. It provides elements for representing facts (expressions) as well as methods of deduction. An application partially based on this model was presented in Section 3.5.2.2.

Other models emerge from the tabular representation of data as in Table 3.3 (Section 3.2) for the introduction to the classification problems (Section 5.1.1.1).

Semantic nets (**knowledge nets**) [148,177,187] have been demonstrated to be more attractive for representing knowledge in semantic analysis (Section 4.4) than the above-mentioned models.

In its simplest form, a semantic net is a set of **nodes**, each node representing a semantic concept. A node may be denoted. In general, undenoted nodes represent complex facts ("extensive carcinoma of the stomach, metastases to the pancreas, the regional lymph nodes, and the omentum"). A node may be connected to another node by a **relation** (Section 5.1). Relations are not necessarily symmetric.

Thus, the object triplet (PATIENT, FINDING, RENAL HEMORRHAGE) is represented as:

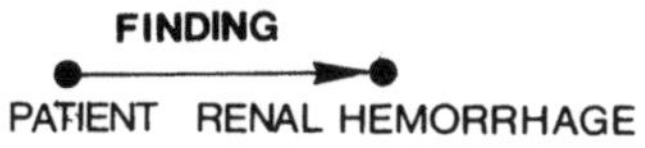

Decomposition of the compound attribute FINDING into the attributes LOC(ation) and MORPH(ology) gives the semantic net:

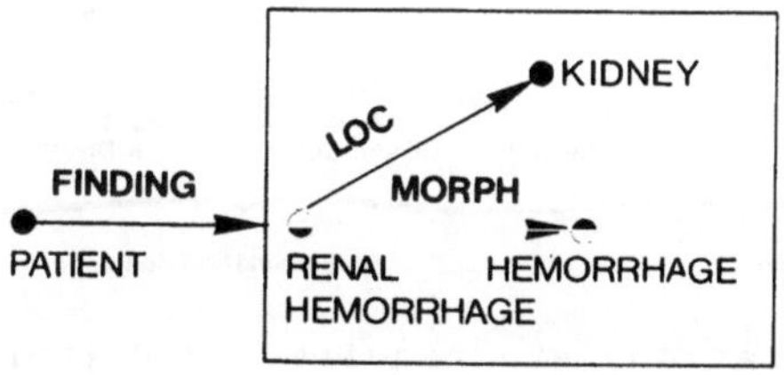

The great flexibility in the definition of nodes and relations allows the representation of complex facts.

"Focal acute inflammation of the kidney" contains a value of the compound attribute "inflammation". This utterance can be represented as:

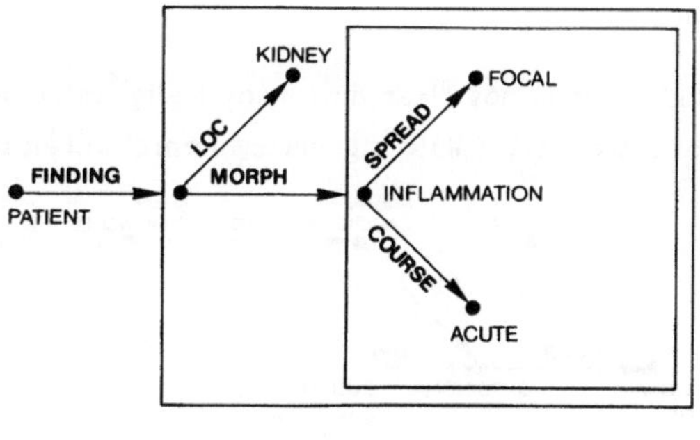

The last two examples illustrate the mapping of the deep structure onto **hierarchic** semantic nets. Each node represents a complex semantic concept, which can be partitioned such that each "node" is itself a semantic net.

The generalization to hierarchic semantic nets corresponds to the recursive definition of object triplets and to a generalization of trees used for representing hierarchic relations (Fig. 3.12, 3.13 in Section 3.4.2.2). In trees the only relation permitted is the hyponymy-relation and each relation points to only one node, whereas in semantic nets each node may be reached by several relations of different type.

Semantic nets are well-suited for relating background knowledge to specific knowledge concerning an observation unit.

If the anatomic structure of the urogenital system is represented as a semantic net, then from "glomerulitis" we may directly deduce an inflammation of the kidney:

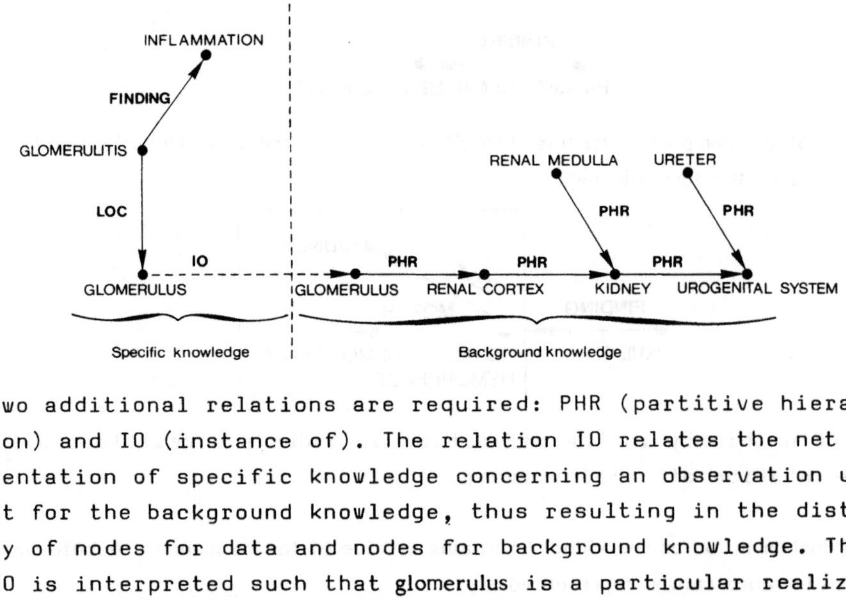

Only two additional relations are required: PHR (partitive hierarchic relation) and IO (instance of). The relation IO relates the net for the representation of specific knowledge concerning an observation unit to the net for the background knowledge, thus resulting in the distinguishability of nodes for data and nodes for background knowledge. The relation IO is interpreted such that glomerulus is a particular realization of the concept glomerulus.

For example, in the following net it is not clear how many malignant tumors are described as long as the relation IO is not introduced (GHR = generic hierarchic relation):

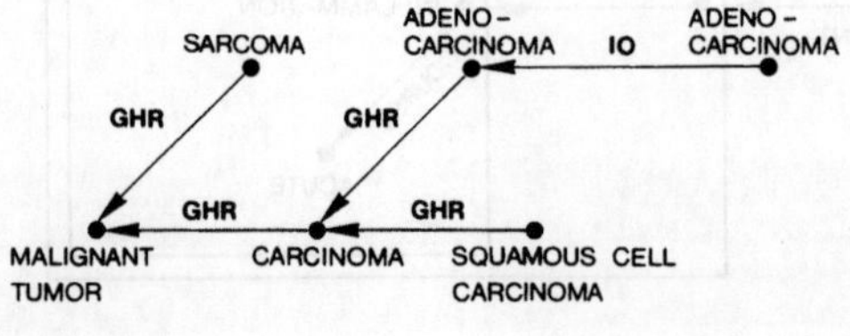

If the relation IO and subsequently the relation GHR is followed until the end of the chain, then a single malignant tumor is found.

Therefore, the relation IO serves for the **activation** of knowledge. If the model "learns" that in an observation unit an adenocarcinoma was found, then the knowledge is activated that it is a carcinoma and a malignant tumor without mentioning these facts explicitly.

Remark: At this point a special problem in access strategy arises. Both parts of the systems knowledge may be connected immediately, i.e., when the specific knowledge is captured or later, when the background knowledge is needed. Systems that immediately build connections are able to answer questions quickly, but face the problem of "combinatorial explosion" when all possible connections are required and nothing is known about what is needed in the future. A system establishing connections only when they are needed, for example, to give an answer, may have intolerably long search times in applications of practical magnitude. The decision about the moment best-suited to establish connections requires a careful analysis of the expected use of such a system.

To assure the correct interpretation of semantic nets, the requirement for the list of values of an attribute must be accomplished (Section 3.1).

Thus, the following net permits different interpretations such as:

- carcinoma of the kidney and inflammation of the liver,
- carcinoma of the liver and inflammation of the kidney,
- carcinoma and inflammation of the liver and the kidney.

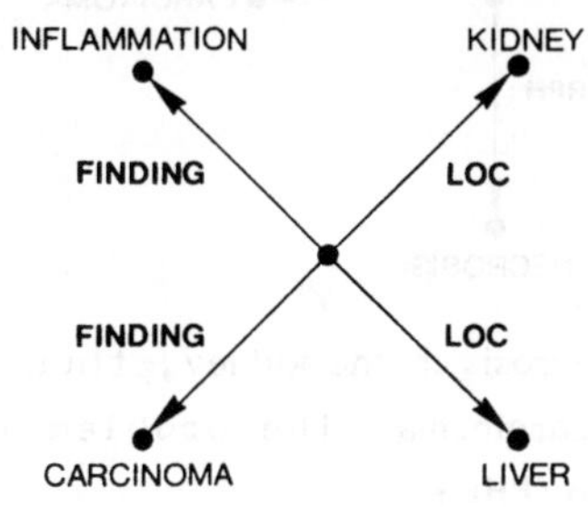

This problem results from the fact that, for example, the attribute LOC can have different values for the observation unit represented in the undenoted node. This must always be excluded in semantic nets, at least if there are relations, which can be combined with each other.

Interpretation is unambiguous only when the morphologic finding and the localization are kept together as a unit to which the relation FINDING points:

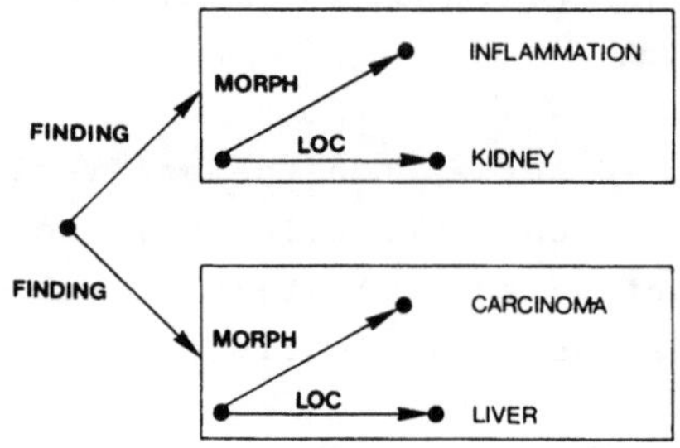

Therefore, the utterance represented in the example describes two findings. In order to make sure that there is always a correct interpretation, even if more relations are added, both findings must be distinguished (e.g., $FINDING_1$ and $FINDING_2$).

To answer a query concerning all locations of pathologic alterations, one follows the relation FINDING and subsequently the relation LOC up to the corresponding node. If all morphologic alterations are required, one follows the relation FINDING and subsequently the relation MORPH up to the corresponding node.

The same problem comes up when necrosis in kidney carcinoma is represented in the following net:

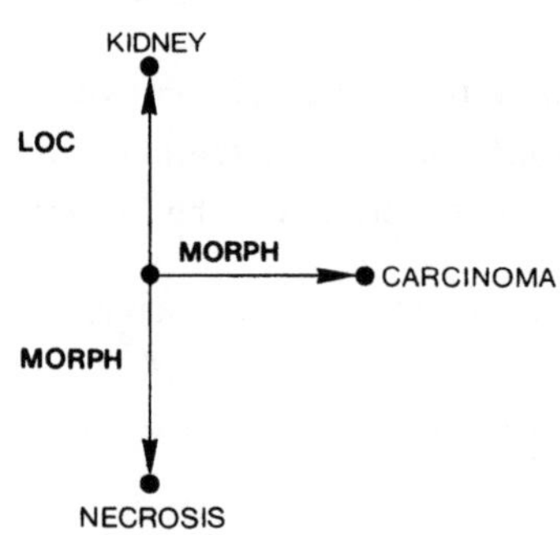

It may be interpreted as necrosis in the kidney, thus pointing to a medical fact other than necrosis in a carcinoma. The problem is resolved by using the previously defined relation PHR:

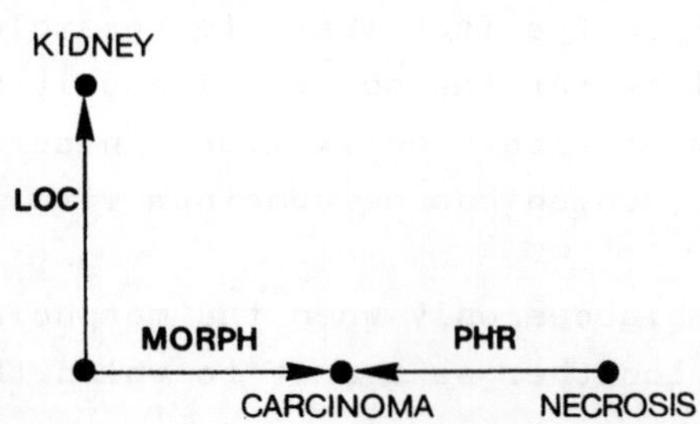

Now, this structure makes clear that necrosis and carcinoma belong together and that this union is located in the kidney.

A semantic net may be extended by additional relations. For example, the utterance pyelonephritis caused by E. coli combined with fever can be represented with the relations MORPH, LOC, FUNC(tion), and ETIO(logy) (Section 5.1.3.7.2):

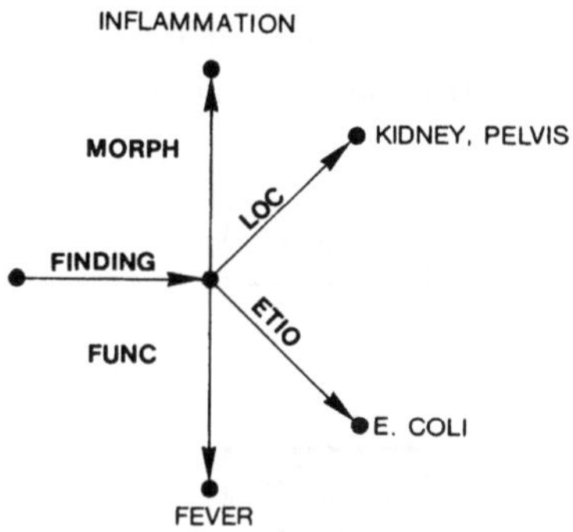

Semantic nets are well-suited for the representation of **pathogenic** relations. This is especially important, because practically none of the common classifications (Section 3.4.5) considers this essential medical relation.

If the relation PATHO is defined, then one gets the following semantic net:

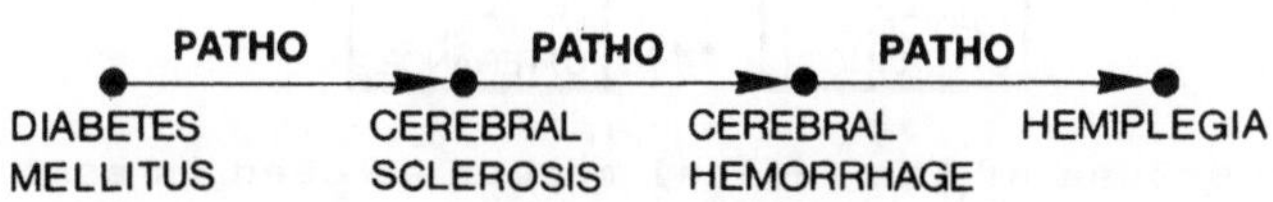

This compressed form can be further extended into a hierarchic semantic net:

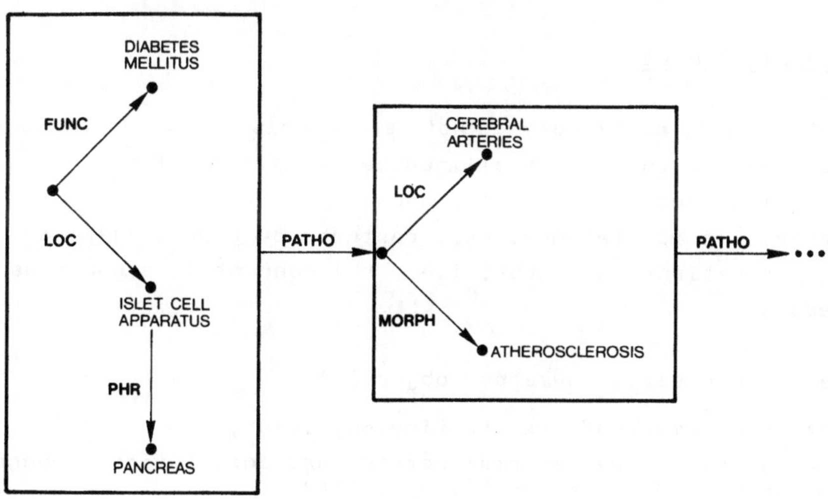

5.1.3 Data Structures in Medicine

In this section, we explain some typical data structures used in medicine. "Typical" means that the structure is either frequently found or it is found in several subfields of medicine. It does not mean that the structure is strictly defined. The sequence of examples is selected to illustrate the recursive nature of the definition of compound objects (Fig. 5.6). The variability of details in the "same" structure illustrates the difficulties in standardization caused by multiple factors.

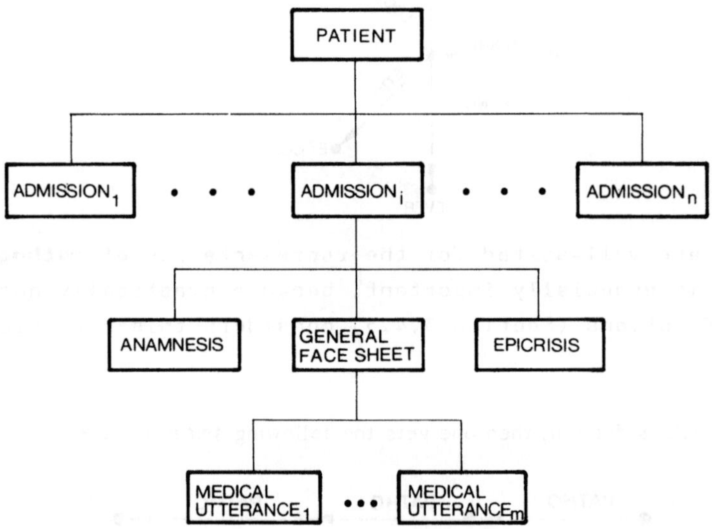

Fig. 5.6: Data structure of the medical record as used in some applications

5.1.3.1 Medical Record

The concept of **medical history** is not used consistently. On the one hand, it is understood as the set of all medically relevant facts during the life of a patient and, on the other hand, it is restricted to the selection of facts, interpretations, etc. captured on paper, film, or other means during a patient encounter, i.e., the concept is synonymous to the **medical record**.

The medical record serves numerous objectives:

- support the memory of the treating physician,
- communication between several persons and institutions engaged in the diagnostic and therapeutic processes,

- document for the justification of execution or omission of manipulations such as diagnostic tests or therapeutic procedures,
- device in medical education,
- protocol in retrospective observational studies,
- document for the management of administrative tasks.

From the medical standpoint, the medical record contains the most general model of a patient. Because of the many individuals adding data to or retrieving data from the medical record, criteria are needed concerning the attributes to be observed as well as their values, codings, and interrelations. But there is no standardization for anyone of these elements that has reached more than local acceptance.

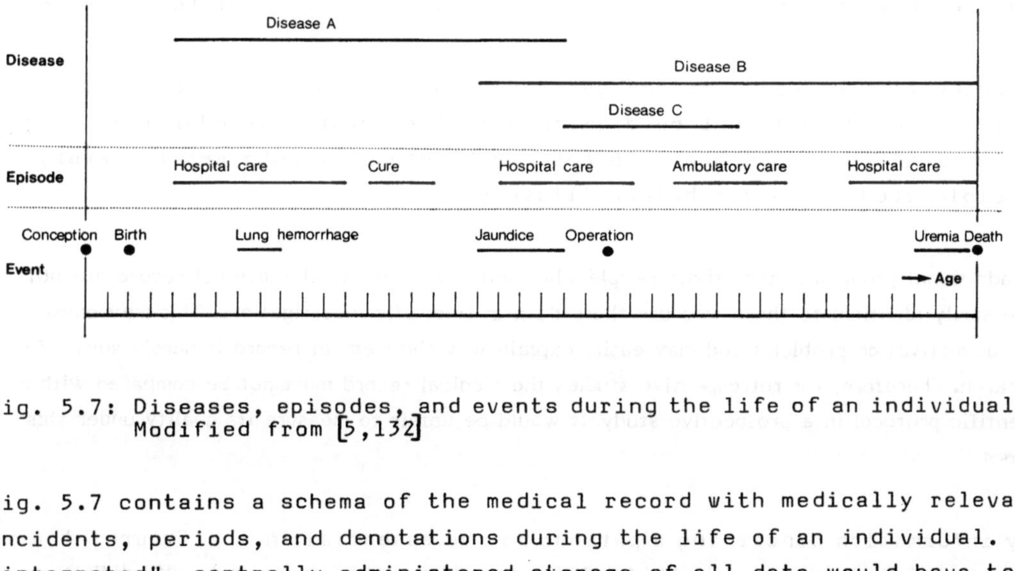

Fig. 5.7: Diseases, episodes, and events during the life of an individual. Modified from [5,132]

Fig. 5.7 contains a schema of the medical record with medically relevant incidents, periods, and denotations during the life of an individual. An "integrated", centrally administered storage of all data would have to include very different data sources such as practicing physicians, ambulatory settings, clinics, and institutions of public health. But multiple legal and technical difficulties stand in the way. Therefore, instead of a single person-oriented medical record, there are at least as many medical records as different institutions serving the patient. Their structure and content depends more on the institution and on the people contributing data to the medical record than on generally accepted models.

Classification of the attributes in the medical record into family history, personal history, present complaints, findings, diagnoses, and epicrisis does not yet result in a sufficiently precise structure, particularly, because not even this classification is generally accepted.

In general, the medical record contains the most voluminous data collected for a patient, but frequently supplies insufficient information. The search for certain data in a medical record, or even the search for all patients with data satisfying certain conditions, is so expensive and unreliable that many physicians engaged in research keep their own files on interesting cases. This adds to the incompleteness of the medical record and to its depreciation.

It probably would be unjustified to state that excessive individualism of physicians or casual attitude towards collection and documentation of data is responsible for the general chaos present in medical record systems. If every possible medical query is admitted, then there is no way to define a concrete model. The number of necessary attributes, values, and relations exceeds every practical limit, because the above-mentioned functions, which reach from a scientific data collection to a file for medical reports, findings, and temperature curves, pose different requirements on the number of attributes and on the completeness of data.

Retrospective studies for the generation of hypotheses, based on the medical record, will not be dismissed in the future. Standardization of the medical record in order to get a complete attribute set for every possible study is nevertheless illusory.

An additional problem is that those people who contribute data to the medical record are not necessarily identical to those who use these data in scientific investigations. This may cause serious motivation problems and may easily explain why the medical record is hardly suited for research. Therefore, for retrospective studies the medical record must not be compared with a scientific protocol in a prospective study. It would be unfair to measure its quality under this aspect.

Any information concerning a patient may be essential in the future; therefore, it has been argued that all data should be captured: "My definition of the medical record is all alphabetic and numeric characters of any meaning to the individual, the patient and the doctor" [4, page 26]. Here medical history and medical record are confused and the difference between data and information is overlooked. As long as a suitable structure for the medical record is missing, the increase of the amount of data is more likely to decrease the quality of information than vice versa.

Insight into this unsatisfactory situation has stimulated attempts and recommendations for improvements [10,24,106,147,162]. These almost always call for additions to the record, which consist of operationally defined attributes to be completely observed (Section 5.1.3.2).

5.1.3.2 General Face Sheet

With the advent of automated support systems in medicine, efforts have been expanded to make the medical record better suited for a fact-oriented evaluation by specific aids (see list in [71]). The best-known result of these efforts in Germany is the "Allgemeiner Krankenblattkopf" [10] (general face sheet).

The recommended attributes are: consecutive medical record number, sex, multiple birth, birth date, name, marital status, address, nationality, paying authority, consecutive number of the general face sheet (for the same patient), admission date, admission reason, class of care, discharge date, discharge type, discharging physician, hospital, diagnoses.

These attributes can be arranged in a structure, which considers the most important relations (Fig. 5.8). The data for the attributes on the first level are invariant during a single hospital stay. Depending on the hospital organization, the attributes on the second level may be observed several times.

For example, this is the case if several hospitals have a common admission facility with a common "admission number". Thus, a patient admitted to the surgery may first be treated in an internal clinic for heart insufficiency. If this corresponds to a new admission and to a new medical record, then a new general face sheet must be filed.

Finally, the attribute diagnoses is subordinated to admission, because there may be several diagnoses during a single hospital stay.

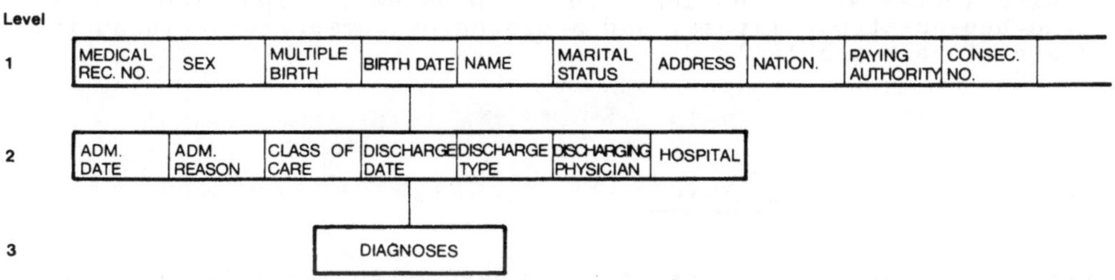

Fig. 5.8: Data structure for the attributes of the general face sheet

The data are used for computation of several medical or administrative parameters such as:

- seasonal variations of disease frequencies (more precisely of the admission frequencies for given diagnoses),

- duration of stay (depending on disease, sex, age, admission reason, ...),
- disease frequencies (depending on sex, age, occupation, ...),
- admission frequencies depending on occupation.

This list of attributes for inpatients is also suited for outpatients. However, documentation in outpatient settings faces even more serious difficulties in organizing the data [117].

5.1.3.3 Problem-Oriented Medical Record

The problem-oriented medical record [175] has been introduced in order to improve patient care as well as education of physicians by grouping the data according to **problems.** The usual chronological recording of data is replaced by the identification of the patients problems and their systematic assignment to diagnosis and therapy. This assignment corresponds to the behavior of the well-experienced physician; it imposes the mental discipline required for the adjustment to the goal of solving the problems.

The problem-oriented medical record consists of the following components:

- **data base** (complaints, findings, social data, present disease, history, laboratory data),
- **problem list** (consecutively numbered past and present problems),
- **treatment plan** (diagnostic and therapeutic manipulations and their assignment to the problems),
- **course** (observations assigned to the problems, "flow diagrams" with time-dependent parameters, and a discharge summary describing the state of each problem).

5.1.3.4 Fundamental Documentation

The term "fundamental documentation" has been established for the storage and retrieval of the data of the general face sheet. The same aspects are present in the discharge summary for inpatients and the encounter form for outpatients. The main ideas underlying the recommendation of the general face sheet are still valid, but technologic development makes some extensions possible. However, in doing this, the understandable desire to observe as many attributes as possible should be treated with caution.

The desires of different clinics or physicians are by no means identical. Therefore, the set of attributes and, consequently, the data volume grows very fast and many attributes are insufficiently defined. The data volume quickly overburdens the data acquisition process, especially when the interest in certain problems decreases. In consequence, data control suffers to the extent that both accuracy and completeness decrease. Workload, increasing error rate, and incompleteness finally result in abandonment of the documentation or in a total shift to documentation personnel.

At present, fundamental documentation is performed in many hospitals, although the underlying data structures differ widely. Common characteristics involve:

- the data structure is identical for all specific medical subfields,
- the attributes are a subset of the attributes constituting the medical record,
- fundamental documentation does not replace a well-defined part of a structured medical record, but is done **additionally**.

From these characteristics several consequences can be drawn:

- data acquisition is retrospective from the medical record,
- data are mostly acquired by special personnel and not by the physician, which is responsible for the medical record,
- there is a (possibly very large) delay between observation of the attributes and data acquisition for fundamental documentation,
- there is frequently no control of relevance and completeness by qualified personnel, especially when data are acquired after discharge of the patient.

Recognition of these consequences protects against some frequent misunderstandings, which may result in serious outcomes. The most important misunderstanding is that more expensive technical equipment, more elegant data acquisition and presentation (e.g., using terminals with direct access to the stored data), and the extension of the attribute set marks the crossing from fundamental documentation to a "hospital information system". There is no such crossing, because the needs of a hospital information system can only be accomplished if data capture and acquisition are organized in a way, which is neither required nor necessary for the fundamental documentation. As long as data are acquired by special personnel in order to keep the physician from changing his habits in recording medical data, and as long as the medical record is insufficiently structured, more expensive methods will have the same problems as the medical record. In addition, they will lose the favorable relation between costs and benefits. Such misunderstandings are well-suited to discredit the methods of information processing in medicine.

However, when the limitations are recognized, there are some possible extensions, which do not complicate the data structure significantly, but make fundamental documentation a valuable tool. If carefully planned and handled, this tool may not only be employed in the creation of tables for speeches or publications, but provide valuable information both for research and patient care (Section 5.1.3.7).

5.1.3.5 Anamnesis

Anamnesis (medical history) is frequently the most important information source in the diagnostic and therapeutic processes [60]. The problems discussed so far with respect to the medical record are most clearly exhibited in anamnesis. The history is usually taken during a conversation between physician and patient ("interview"). This analogy with other situations, such as public opinion poll-taking, easily misleads us into thinking that techniques well tested in these situations may be applied equally well in medical history taking. But this creates several difficulties:

- In a public opinion poll and in an epidemiologic poll the hypotheses, the relations among attributes and hypotheses, and the values of the attributes are defined and their number is low. In the anamnesis in general, the set of hypotheses is open and one of the objectives is to reduce this set, in other words, to reach the state that is given, a priori, in a poll.
- In a poll two partners on the same level participate. In anamnesis, both partners have very distinct roles: the patient is seeking health and the physician is offering help.
- Because of gaps in the patient's memory or intentional omissions, anamnesis is not like questioning with a definite end. Questions arising during the diagnostic or therapeutic process may always initiate a continuation of the anamnesis.
- The goal of anamnesis is to elucidate the individual problems of the patient. This results in a conflict situation for the physician. He has to find and treat the causes of the patients complaints and he must not overlook anything "important". That is, he has to find a disturbance even if the patient does not complain about it. The first goal needs an anamnesis strictly concentrated on the - unknown - outcome and the skipping of bypaths. The second goal needs completeness. This discrepancy of elucidation and treatment of individual complaints, on the one hand, and of health checkups, on the other hand, is of growing importance in medicine.
- Anamnesis not only captures information but also serves to establish a confidential relationship between patient and physician. In addition, it may have the function of education and psychologic relief (katharsis).

Therefore, anamnesis has no detailed structure of general validity. "Standardization" of compound attributes, which have frequently been attempted in internal medicine [58,61,101], do not replace operational definitions necessary for computer support. Moreover, many physicians question the desirability of abandoning the human dialog because of its nonformalizable functions [58].

Computer support may be indicated in two special situations:

- **General overview** by questions covering a broad spectrum of diseases in order to reduce the set of possible diseases, i.e., to get indications to diseases or to exclude diseases of vital importance (asking for leading symptoms). This situation arises primarily in health screening, the volume of which is steadily growing. It is here where in any case physicians may be replaced for other reasons (Section 1.1).
- **Special anamnesis** as decision support in a strictly-defined differential diagnosis.

A general overview already demands a voluminous questionnaire [34,101]. The method of processing depends mainly on the type of questions, i.e., whether the possible answers are predetermined ("closed" questions, multiple-choice principle) or not ("open" questions). The most restrictive type of closed questions permits only the answers "yes" and "no". But experience has shown [152] that at least the answers "do not know" and "please explain" should be provided.

The first level of standardization consists of the enumeration of possible questions and answers. All questions are put to the patient in a fixed sequence (Fig. 5.9).

The best-known catalog of this type, no doubt, is the Cornell Medical Index Health Questionnaire [22] containing 195 questions.

Typically, when these questionnaires are compared with a human dialog, they provide more complete data with respect to general findings and less complete data with respect to details. This fact is not at all surprising, because anamnesis is a special sequential decision problem (Section 3.5).

Consequently, the next level of "standardization" [101] is the employment of a model for decision support. The predicate logic model results in a hierarchic questionnaire, where each answer is assigned a "branching address" pointing to the next question to be asked (Fig. 5.10).

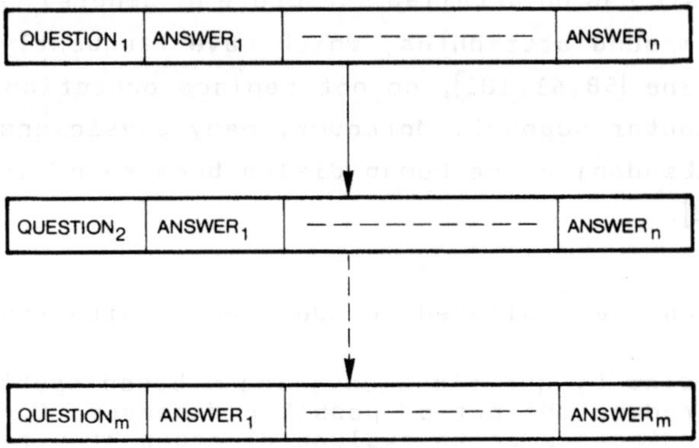

Fig. 5.9: Structure of a linear questionnaire. Each QUESTION may have $ANSWER_1$ to $ANSWER_n$

For example, detailed questions concerning type, localization, and frequency of pain can be skipped if an "initial" question for pain has been denied.

Processing open questions is much more difficult than closed questions and requires the employment of linguistic methods (Chapter 4).

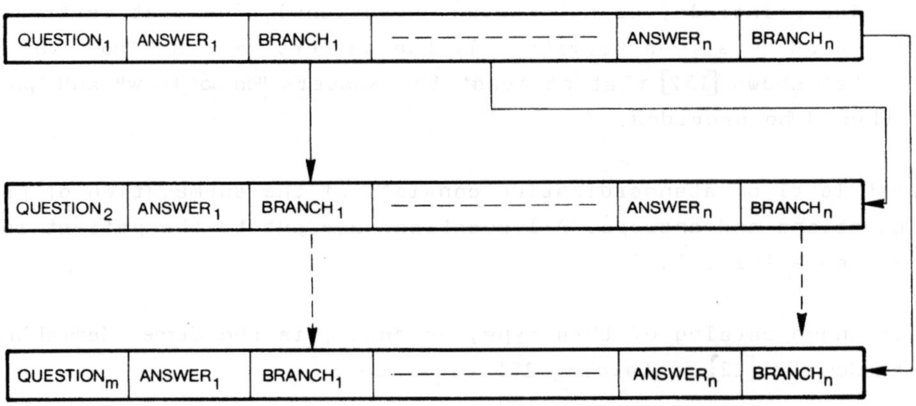

Fig. 5.10: Structure of a hierarchic questionnaire

5.1.3.6 Epicrisis

Epicrisis is the completion of the medical record and presents a summary and a judgement of the course of a disease. It is practically identical with the medical report (Section 5.5.1.1). There are no general agreements concerning content and structure of the epicrisis.

In [17] the following structure is proposed (optional parts are parenthesized):

patient identification
treatment period
diagnoses
(differential diagnoses)
(admission reason)
(admission state)
(discharge state)
therapy
(course, complications, adverse reactions)
discharge type
treatment outcomes
prognosis.

In each particular case, the content will mainly depend on the individual situation, especially when secretarial resources are restricted or the medical report is significantly delayed.

5.1.3.7 Medical Utterance

This compound object contains four objects (Fig. 5.11): What has been observed (ATTRIBUTE), in whom (PATIENT), when (TIME), and by whom (SOURCE). ATTRIBUTE may contain just the value or also a denotation of the attribute itself (Section 5.1.2.2). The objects PATIENT and ATTRIBUTE correspond to the object triplet.

PATIENT	ATTRIBUTE	TIME	SOURCE

Fig. 5.11: Structure of a medical utterance

Relations among different realizations of such an object are of formal or semantic type. The most important **formal** relations are based on the equality of data in different realizations, like:

- PATIENT: all utterances concerning the same patient,
- ATTRIBUTE: all patients, in which the same attribute (with the same outcome) has been observed,
- PATIENT and ATTRIBUTE: longitudinal studies,
- TIME and SOURCE: all services of a medical unit at a given time.

The basic model in Fig. 5.11 can be structured in more detail according to the needs of special domains.

In general, coding of TIME will present no serious difficulties. Usually a calendar date suffices; if necessary, the time may be added (observation of time-dependent attributes, e.g., daily glucose profile). In some applications TIME is needed twice (begin/end of validity of an utterance).

The SOURCE is a hospital (as in the ATTRIBUTE "transfer from"), a medical unit (as ECG-unit), an administrative unit (as admission unit), a physician, etc. Mostly, these data can easily be coded.

The patient identification PATIENT (Section 5.1.3.7.1) causes more difficulties, as also the ATTRIBUTE (medical information, Section 5.1.3.7.2).

5.1.3.7.1 Patient Identification

In the simplest case, patient identification PATIENT is numerically coded. Criteria for the quality of coding are:

- **redundancy** (number of digits or occupancy density),
- identification degree, especially
  - **selectivity** (probability that different patients receive different codes),
  - **specifity** (probability that the same patient receives the same code at different admissions),
- **self-generability** (derivation of the code from characteristics of the patient).

There is extensive literature on the identification problem (e.g., [169]), a fact which points to the relevance of a practical solution. Without such a solution, the linkage of data and patients is insufficiently safe.

The advantage of consecutively **assigned** codes, like medical record number, is the low redundancy (minimum code length for a given number of patients). But there are gaps with a non-neglectable frequency, when the codes are assigned through a manual procedure (i.e., unoccupied codes, which makes control of completeness difficult) or even doublets (the same code is assigned to different patients). Frequency of both cases can amount to up to 2% depending on the quality of the admission unit. Another advantage of consecutive numbers is that they can always be assigned, even for unconscious patients. These advantages are balanced by the disadvantage that hardly anybody is able to remember such numbers. The necessary costly file search for a number during patient readmission carries additional error risk, resulting in different numbers for the same patient at different times. Moreover, the linkage of data from different sources with independent codes is impossible. This problem is well-known in many clinics with separate admission units for each individual hospital.

The previously mentioned difficulties are more easily overcome when the code is **generated** from identifying attributes of a patient. The disadvantage is the redundancy, i.e., the prolongation of the code. Generated codes are more easily remembered, but they require information from the patient (not available from an unconscious patient!). The authors of the "allgemeiner Krankenblattkopf" (Section 5.1.3.2) have proposed a 9-digit **ID-number**, consisting of the birth date, one digit for the sex, and a 2-digit numeric code for the name (maiden name) [170].

If the attributes coded in the ID-number are independent and uniformly distributed, then the number of possible ID-numbers is

$$365 \cdot 100 \cdot 2 \cdot 100 = 7.3 \cdot 10^6 .$$

The actual deviation from a Uniform Distribution and the application of combinatorial rules give an idea on the relatively high probability of the same ID-number in different patients. Several investigations [170] resulted in about 65 doublets among 20,000 patients.

In a recent publication [45] it was found that for a data base with 137,474 patients the probability of hitting an already existing ID-number is about 5%. The data base contained 1,726 doublets, 47 triplets, and 1 quadruplet.

A way out is a general **personal identification number**. But the simplification of data linkage resulting from such a number is exactly the reason for political objections against its introduction.

The risk of a false assignment due to misspellings in the identification number can be reduced only by an increase of redundancy. In numeric codes this is done mostly by adding a **check character**.

If the code number is $n = n_m n_{m-1} \ldots n_1$, and the ordered character set $C = \{c_1, c_2, \ldots, c_k\}$, then the check character p is

$$p = c_j, \quad \text{with } j = \sum_{i=1}^{m} i \cdot n_i \text{ modulo } k \quad (k > m) .$$

For example, if the character set C consists of the digits 0 to 9 ($c_1=0$, $c_2=1$, . . . , $c_{10}=9$), and if n = 32,745, then

$$j = \sum_{i=1}^{5} i \cdot n_i \text{ modulo } 10 = 5+8+21+8+15 \text{ modulo } 10 = 57 \text{ modulo } 10 = 7,$$

and the **check digit** $p = c_7$ is equal to 6.

Frequently in medical data processing, the patient identification has to be extended by a compound attribute consisting of the name, birth date (if not part of the code), and maiden name.

5.1.3.7.2 Medical Information

In the "allgemeiner Krankenblattkopf" (Section 5.1.3.2) this object is identical to the set of diagnoses. But documentation is significantly improved when symptoms, signs, and procedures are added. The last object is especially important for surgical units. In addition, relations have to be considered. They account for the extension of the chronological list of medical utterances to a semantic net (Section 5.1.2.3) and require a structure of a medical utterance like the one in Fig. 5.12. This structure permits data acquisition in prospective studies and in experiments ("controlled clinical trials").

The structure in Fig. 5.12 is also applicable to the problem-oriented medical record (Section 5.1.3.3). "Data base" and "problem list" correspond to a list of medical utterances. The "treatment plan" corresponds to a list of therapeutic/diagnostic procedures with the respective relations. The course of a "case" can be represented by considering the TIME. Therefore, the data structure is a base for the description of the medical decision process.

SNOMED [33] (Section 3.4.5.4) has presented a "nomenclature" with a semantic structure, which determines a structure of medical information useful in many areas of medicine (Fig. 5.13).

The complete structure of a medical information is modified according to the needs of special applications.

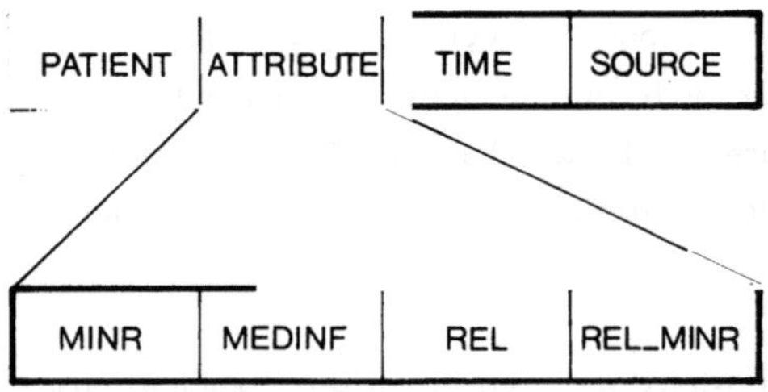

Fig. 5.12: Structure of a medical utterance when relations are considered. The denotations are:

MINR: consecutive number of the medical utterance,

MEDINF: medical information (diagnosis, therapy, sign, symptom),

REL: relation to the medical utterance number REL_MINR

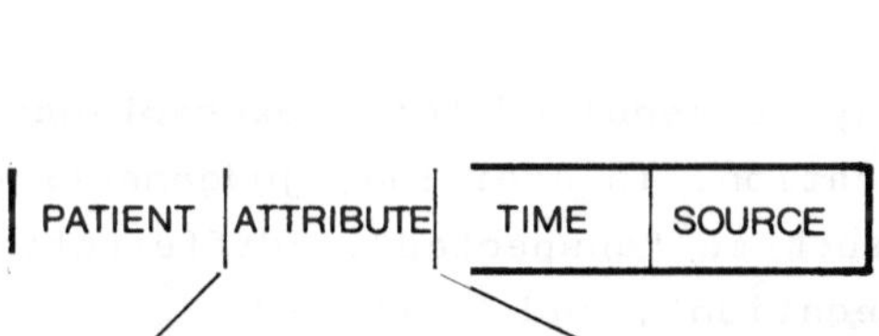

Fig. 5.13: Structure of a medical utterance based on the structure of a medical information due to SNOMED [33] (S=certainty, P=procedures, R=result, D=diseases, T=topography, M=morphology, E=etiology, F=function)

Utterances in **pathology** require the dimensions T, M, and E. In **clinical pathology** dimension F is additionally needed. If the method of specimen collection or the type of examination is required, then dimension P is needed.

In **microbiology/bacteriology** dimensions P, T, M, and E are used.

In the **clinical laboratory** dimensions P (specimen collection and type of examination) and M (results) are required. There are different opinions with respect to dimension M. One opinion is that the laboratory has to produce results and has to refrain from every diagnostic evaluation. The other opinion is that reliable evaluation of the result demands diagnostic evaluation in the laboratory.

In **clinical medicine** all dimensions are used in various combinations.

There are two fundamental relations in the basic structure between dimension P and the other dimensions depending on the content of P. One relation is "therapy for", the other one is "examination results in". As a nomenclature, SNOMED does not contain the values of many diagnostic attributes. Because it is appropriate for most problems to acquire not only the interpretation of a test result, but to acquire also the result itself, the object "procedure" (P) must be complemented by a "result" (R) (Fig. 5.13).

Specific additions may be required for **prescriptions** such as frequency and dosage of a medication. In addition, judgements of a medical information may be needed such as "suspected", "differential diagnosis", "certainty", "explicit negation", and "risk of".

Within the semantic dimensions of SNOMED there are many explicit relations and substructures represented in the code. Two examples from morphology, especially important for practical applications, shall be explained (Section 3.1.1).

The concepts of "inflammations" (Fig. 3.13 in Section 3.4.2.2) are described by the orthogonal attributes "course", "spread", and "circulation alteration" (Table 5.2). The concepts of "neoplasms" are described by the orthogonal attributes "behavior", "differentiation", and "spread" (Table 5.3).

Course	**Spread**	**Circulation alteration**
acute	focal	serous
subacute	diffuse	exudative
chronic	multifocal	fibrinous
...	...	...

Table 5.2: Orthogonal attributes for the description of "inflammations" according to SNOMED [33]

Behavior	Differentiation	Spread
benign	well differentiated	in situ
malignant	moderately differentiated	primary
	poorly differentiated	metastatic
	undifferentiated	

Table 5.3: Orthogonal attributes for the description of "neoplasms" according to SNOMED [33]

Necessity and problems of a detailed data structure are even more clear for clinical signs and symptoms, because they have often multiple and rarely operationally defined relations to diagnoses and therapies [53].

5.1.3.7.3 Relations

Besides the relations embedded in the structure of the compound attributes, there are many relations among objects whose relevance depends on the application, and which have to be explicitly represented. Relations of very general relevance for the representation of medical information involve:

- "therapy" **for** "diagnosis",
- "diagnosis" **complicates** "diagnosis" or "therapy",
- "diagnosis" or "finding" is an **adverse reaction** due to "therapy",
- "examination" **results** in "finding".

An **adverse reaction** (due to a therapy) is an unwanted event, the conditional probability of which is greater than its probability in the population due to a causal dependence. The notion of **complication** is used in two ways. It is either interpreted as an adverse reaction due to a therapy (infection of a surgical wound; bone marrow alterations caused by treatment with cytostatics) or as a consequence in the course of a disease, i.e., a pathogenic chain (perforation of the stomach due to gastric ulcer).

The following utterances may be part of a medical record:

20.1.78 Begin of a therapy with corticoids for acute ulcerative colitis.
5.3.78 Emergency admission due to treatment-caused perforated gastric ulcer.
5.3.78 Suture of the defect.
6.3.78 Therapy with cephalosporin for beginning peritonitis.
20.3.78 Discharge after healing.

MINR	TIME	P	D	T	M	E	F	REL	REL_MINR	Text
1	20.1.78			T67000	M41030	E8510				Colon, acute ulcerative inflammation, corticoids
2	5.3.78	P0030		T63000	M38000			N	1	Emergency admission, stomach, ulcer
3	5.3.78			T63230	M14700			C	2	Gastric wall, perforation
4	5.3.78	P1600		T63230				Th	3	Suture, gastric wall
5	6.3.78			TY4400	M40000	E7216		C	3	Peritoneum, inflammation, cephalosporin
6	20.3.78	P0100					F02450			Discharge, healed

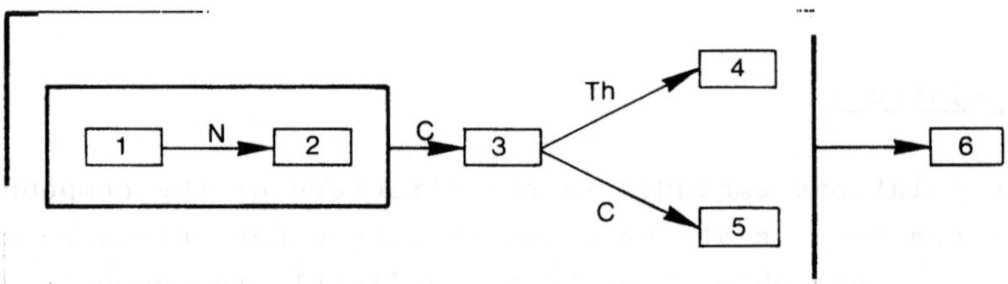

Fig. 5.14: Tabular representation and semantic net of a formalized medical record. For the structure of a medical information see Fig. 5.13. Relations (REL): N=adverse reaction, C=complication, Th=therapy for

This results in a formally representable medical record based on the structure of SNOMED (Fig. 5.14). The explicit relations point in unit no. 2 to an adverse reaction due to no. 1, in unit no. 3 to a complication of unit no. 2, and in unit no. 5 to a complication of unit no. 3. The relation "Th" marks unit no. 4 as the therapy for unit no. 3.

5.2 Data Acquisition and Input

Data acquisition may be divided into three phases.

Data capture is the observation of the attributes and results in rough data recorded in a protocol. **Data preparation** transfers the rough data into the form required in the data base. For example, coding and simple arithmetic computations are included in this phase (computation of relative frequencies for white blood count). Usually, the results are again transcribed. Finally, the prepared data are transformed to a computer-readable **medium** such as punch cards or paper tape (**data fixation**).

5.2.1 Organizational Structures

We introduce the above-mentioned working routines by an organizational structure frequently found in medical record storage and retrieval (Table 5.4).

Phase	Source	Acquirer	Data storage
data capture	patient/specimen	physician/nurse	medical record
data preparation	medical record	documentation personnel	keypunch data sheet
data fixation	keypunch data sheet	card puncher	punch card

Table 5.4: Organization of data acquisition in medical record storage and retrieval, from [85]

The medical record contains rough data as well as prepared data (Section 5.1.3.1). Documentation personnel convert these data into update records for the data base, prepared and recorded on keypunch data sheets (Fig. 5.15). These data sheets serve as a model for transferring the data to a computer readable medium.

The most important criteria for judging the organization of data acquisition are actuality, reliability, and costs. They are strongly interrelated.

Actuality is a measure of the time from the origin of a datum in an observation unit to its storage in the data base. **Reliability** is a measure of the probability that a datum in the data base is correct. The **costs** of data acquisition include the costs for observation, preparation, and fixation of the data, as well as for checks and corrections. In the strictest sense, the "costs" caused by false data in the data base have also to be considered. But, because these costs usually cannot be measured, they are frequently neglected, although they may exceed all other costs.

The different organizational forms are classified by means of the **location** of the phases and the degree of **integration**.

The organization of data acquisition represented in Table 5.4 may be characterized as follows: in earlier phases data capture is less well-defined operationally, requires better medically qualified acquirers, and data are more actual and reliable. But this organization is expensive with respect to personnel and time, and it is unreliable.

Reliability is strongly influenced by the design of a data form. Important aspects are the structure of compound attributes, frequencies of attribute values, logical relations between values of different attributes (dependence, independence), code lengths, coding of missing data, and observation order of the attributes.

Data forms include the keypunch data sheet, the mark sense form, and the optical character reader form.

A **keypunch data sheet** (Fig. 5.15) is a mapping of one or more punch cards. Each square corresponds to a column of a punch card. Therefore, the squares are numbered and contain a digit, a letter, or a special character. Additional media for primary data recording are magnetic tape and magnetic disk.

Clinical Trial of MIRACULIN Versus OCULTAN
Data From Patients With Glaucoma Acutum Congestivum

1.	Consecutive number	1	0 1
2.	Therapy (OCULTAN = 1, MIRACULIN = 2)	3	1
3.	Medical record number	4	0 9 3 5 6 8
4.	Admission date	10	1 8 1 1 6 8
5.	Birth date	16	1 5 0 3 9 4
6.	Sex (male = 1, female = 2)	22	2
7.	Height in cm	23	1 6 8
8.	Weight in kg	26	0 7 5
9.	Blood pressure in mm Hg at admission: systolic	29	2 2 5
10.	Blood pressure in mm Hg at admission: diastolic	32	1 3 0

Fig. 5.15: Detail from a keypunch data sheet for data acquisition [64]

Organization is improved by merging different phases (Table 5.4). There are several possibilities for this **integration** [85]:

- The "keypunch data sheet" for data preparation is replaced by a computer readable form, and separate data fixation is omitted. Such computer readable forms involve mark sense forms and optical character reader forms.

In **mark sense forms** fixed positions may be marked by a stroke. Mark sense readers can "read" these marks. Because only the two levels "marked" and "not marked" are possible, each attribute must be converted into a set of binary attributes (Section 3.1.2). This can result in very unclear forms causing high error rates [180]. But, because mark sense forms are cheap, they are frequently used for data fixation.

Optical character reader forms have to be written on typewriters with special types (OCR = Optical Character Reader). Some devices can also read marks, like mark sense form readers, as well as handwritten digits and a few handwritten characters.

- The "keypunch data sheet" for data preparation is replaced by a **prompt** on a terminal (Fig. 5.16). Hence again, separate data fixation is omitted. An immediate check for errors by a computer program is possible, and the delay between data fixation and data input is omitted. Therefore, the data base can be more actual and reliable. A disadvantage is the higher expense of the equipment needed.

- Those parts of the medical record, which are to be acquired, are directly input into a **prompt** on a terminal during data capture. Hence again, separate data preparation and fixation is omitted.

There are additional possibilities for the acquisition of data generated by technical devices [121] (Section 6.1):

- Data are directly transferred from the device to computer readable means (punch card, paper tape, magnetic tape, ...) and are subsequently input without manual data transmission. This is a relatively simple technical solution. Its advantage is that the availability of the device is independent of the availability of the computer, but its disadvantage is the possibly large delay between origin of the data and their checking for errors.

- Data are input directly to the computer or by means of an "interface". This solution needs a more complex technology, but its advantage is, that special computer programs may directly check the data.

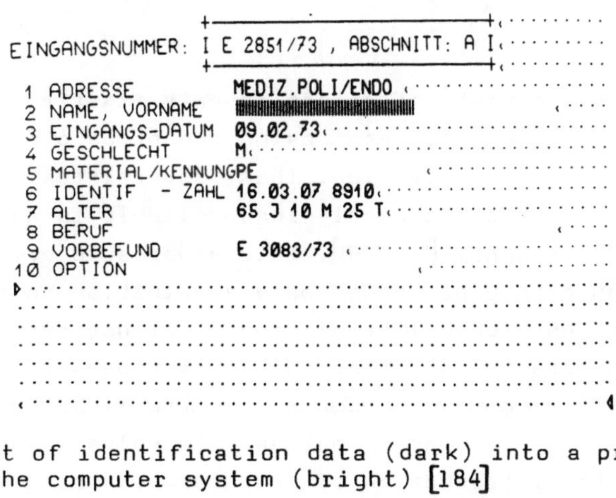
EINGANGSNUMMER: I E 2851/73 , ABSCHNITT: A I

1 ADRESSE MEDIZ.POLI/ENDO
2 NAME, VORNAME [redacted]
3 EINGANGS-DATUM 09.02.73
4 GESCHLECHT M
5 MATERIAL/KENNUNGPE
6 IDENTIF - ZAHL 16.03.07 8910
7 ALTER 65 J 10 M 25 T
8 BERUF
9 VORBEFUND E 3083/73
10 OPTION

Fig. 5.16: Input of identification data (dark) into a prompt projected by the computer system (bright) [184]

With respect to the **localization** of data generation, **centralized** and **decentralized** organization is distinguished. Data capture is usually decentralized. It is impossible to make general statements, whether or not data input should be centralized. Decentralized data input allows a more complete integration of the data acquisition, leading to an improvement in actuality and reliability, whereas centralized data acquisition usually facilitates data linkage. Decentralized data input is not always possible. For example, data preparation may require specific knowledge to such an extent that the necessary personnel is available only in a central unit.

5.2.2 Error Control

The definition of "errors" is much more difficult than may be supposed at first glance. The notion ranges from human mistakes to various statistical errors (error first and second kind in statistical tests, random error, systematic error, ...). An illustrative collection of error sources for medical data is contained in [167].

Errors in **data capture** arise from misinterpretation or defective technical equipment. The most frequent errors occur perhaps in anamnestic data [35,191], especially when calendar dates of events that took place a long time ago are required, or when psychologic factors play an important role, as in facts frequently considered as discriminating (hereditary diseases, epileptic seizures, psychiatric problems).

Non-operationally defined compound attributes are particularly well-suited for **misinterpretation** (percussion, palpation, psychiatric examinations). In different investigations, error frequencies between 15% and 50% are cited [167].

The next major group consists of errors in **data fixation** and **data input**. Here the influence of the data form design cannot be overestimated. Another important factor is motivation. Thus, several tests have illustrated that physicians are frequently less reliable in data acquisition than documentation personnel [76,180]. This experience competes with the postulation to keep data capture and data acquisition in the same hand in order to reduce the probability of transmission errors. Furthermore, it points to the necessity for offering a direct pay-off for every type of data fixation (for example, data acquisition is much more reliable when it is used for a scientific paper). Yet the problem is not easy to solve, and it did not arise solely with the introduction of computer-supported methods.

Transmission errors and **misspellings** are frequently found in numbers, intrinsically. This is a serious problem in laboratory data and identification codes. These errors may cause the misattribution of findings and can result in aggravating secondary errors. Examination of laboratory data suggests that a conventional laboratory experiences an error rate on the order of magnitude of 10% [18].

Systematic investigations have also illustrated how unreliable some data in medical records may be. Thus, [76] reports 1,022 medical records, in which 2/3 failed to record the diagnoses in the right place; every medical record omitted some data. An interesting example of **virtual** data is recorded in [167]: among 575 medical records for readmitted patients in 1/3 of the cases a certain datum was not revaluated, as it should have been, but merely transcribed from the first admission.

Coding errors are more frequent when a larger and a less systematized dictionary is used.

The great spectrum of errors in the **design of trials** may only be mentioned here [85]. They frequently result directly in false conclusions and account for a great share of the "scientific" disagreements.

It is impossible to make general statements about the consequences of errors. They depend on the type and the severity of an error, its influence on decisions, and on the degree of redundancy. In any case, considerable risks arise by the cumulation of errors with respect to a single patient as well as to samples in statistical tests. Frequently, the costs of a subsequent correction are so high, measured in time, money, and difficulty, that control and correction is omitted, even if data are suspected to be false.

The majority of errors occurs before data processing in the strict sense. Therefore, much attention should be paid to the reliability during this phase, particularly, because many errors cannot even later be recognized.

5.2.2.1 <u>Error Detection and Error Supposition</u>

Besides the precautions for the omission of errors, medical informatics is particularly interested in algorithms for error control. This problem may be formulated as a classification problem (Chapter 3):

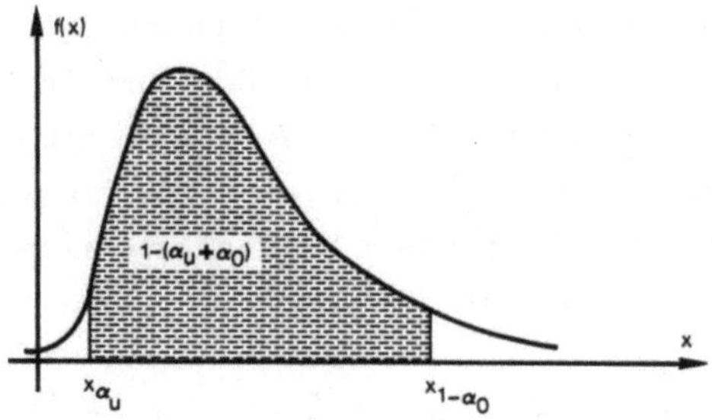

Fig. 5.17: Definition of a 1-dimensional critical region containing a realization with probability $\alpha_u+\alpha_o$. The "normal" region is hatched

Data are observed for a vector $\mathbf{X}$ of attributes. $\mathbf{X}$ defines a k-dimensional space R. The values observed in an observation unit are a realization $\mathbf{x}$ of $\mathbf{X}$. Let $\tilde{R}$ be a subspace of R and $\alpha = P(\mathbf{X} \in \tilde{R})$.

When $\alpha=0$, $\mathbf{x}$ "must" contain an error if $\mathbf{x} \in \tilde{R}$ (**error detection**). When α is smaller than a given α_0, an error is **supposed** if $\mathbf{x} \in \tilde{R}$ (**runaway**).

The methods for error control (**plausibility check**) are classified according to the number of dimensions of $\tilde{R}$, and whether they serve for error detection or for error supposition. In general, one proceeds as in a statistical test with the null hypothesis

H_0: The data vector $\mathbf{x}$ is free of errors.

The **critical region** $\tilde{R}$ is chosen such that the event $\{\mathbf{X} \in \tilde{R}\}$ has a small (given) probability, when H_0 is true and a possibly large probability, when H_0 is not true. The percentiles are estimated from a random sample, because the distribution of $\mathbf{X}$ is in general unknown.

5.2.2.1.1 Univariate Methods

Error detection in case of a 1-dimensional critical region means that x is not a value of attribute X. This class of methods includes in particular: syntactic control (check for admitted structure of a message, e.g., only digits), control of completeness (missing data), control versus extreme values, and control of spelling (particularly in texts).

For **error supposition** one starts from the probability density and defines a critical region (Fig. 5.17):

$$\tilde{R} = \left\{x \,\middle|\, x < x_{\alpha_u} \vee x > x_{1-\alpha_o}\right\}.$$

The probability of error supposition in a correct datum ("error first kind") is at most $\alpha=\alpha_u+\alpha_o$. The region between x_{α_u} and $x_{1-\alpha_o}$ is frequently called **normal region**. In practice, α_u and α_o are given and the respective percentiles are estimated by the empirical percentiles.

5.2.2.1.2 Multivariate Methods

Conceptually, the univariate methods can be directly generalized to multivariate methods.

Examples for error detection are checking of agreement between sex and disease ("carcinoma of the prostate gland" in women) or between age and disease ("scarlatina" in an 80 year old patient). That is, "natural" redundancy is utilized. Redundancy may also artificially be generated for error control (acquisition of the age in addition to admission date and birth date or generation of check characters, see Section 5.1.3.7.1).

Frequently, data supposed to be false are determined in the k-dimensional case by computing a k-dimensional sphere such that the sphere contains the rate (1-α) of the data. The data outside this sphere are then checked. The method is improved for different variances in the different dimensions by computing a k-dimensional ellipsoid, the main axes of which are proportional to the (empirical) variances.

In case of complex distributions, the frequency distribution may be estimated as follows: a distance function is defined and for each observation unit (represented as a point in the k-dimensional attribute space) a value d_n is determined such that exactly n neighbors have a distance not greater than d_n. If d_n exceeds a certain limit, then an error is supposed [46].

The three "different" methods can be subsumed under the same technique:

> A distance function is defined (Euclidean distance, proportional to the inverse of the empirical variance, or some arbitrary function). A sphere is computed around a center containing all points, which have a distance of not more than a limit d. When the center is the gravity center of the data, each data point outside the sphere is supposed to be false; when the center is an observation unit of the sample, the data are supposed to be false, if the value d becomes too large, d defined such that a given number of neighbors fall into the sphere.

It should be kept in mind, that the more careful control of those data, which are supposed to be false, cause an inhomogeneity in the thourough-ness of data observation, an effect that should be avoided in samples

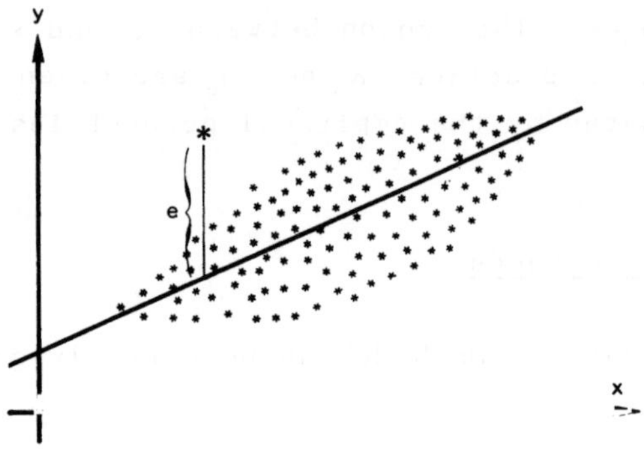

Fig. 5.18: Linear regression analysis for error control

drawn for later statistical analysis.

Because multivariate methods are frequently very extensive, several techniques are employed to reduce the problem to a univariate problem. For example, the principal component analysis (Section 3.3.1.1.3) can serve this purpose. In the extreme case, the analysis results in a few random variables representing the random error with a sufficiently small variance. When the realization of this random variable for an observation unit differs too much from zero, an error is supposed.

The same principle is used when functional **dependences** between attributes are utilized. Thus, a dependence between quantitative attributes can often be employed successfully for error control. If an attribute Y is functionally dependent on a vector $\mathbf{X} = (X_1, X_2, \ldots, X_k)$,

$$Y = f(\mathbf{X}) + E,$$

with the random error E, then the parameters of the function f may be estimated by regression analysis. According to $E = Y - f(\mathbf{X})$, the problem of simultaneous error control for the attribute set $\{Y, X_1, X_2, \ldots, X_k\}$ is reduced to a 1-dimensional problem for E.

This principle is schematically represented in Fig. 5.18 by means of a linear dependence between two attributes X and Y:

$$Y = \underbrace{a \cdot X + b}_{f(X)} + E \quad \text{or} \quad E = Y - a \cdot X - b .$$

The point marked by an asterisk reveals no peculiarities when the dimensions X and Y are analyzed in isolation. But an error is supposed as soon as both attributes are analyzed simultaneously, i.e., as soon as the realization of E is computed.

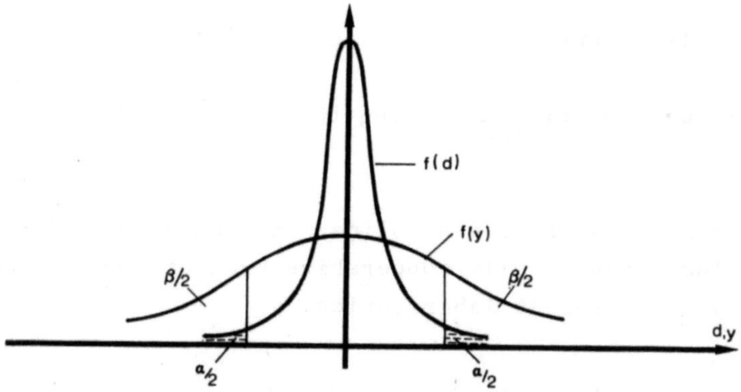

Fig. 5.19: Probability densities of the intraindividual difference D_t between two observations made with distance t and of the interindividual difference Y for the same attribute

Dependent attributes are also found in dependent samples. Particularly important in practice is the **natural block** [85], e.g., when an attribute is observed at different times in the same observation unit. This fact is especially useful in the clinical laboratory for error control.

A practical application in controlling result attribution has been described in [122].

Let X_t be a random variable, representing an attribute X for a patient at time t. From the data collected during the past year, realizations of the intraindividual random variables $D_a=X_a-X_{a+t}$ are computed (i.e., a is the time of the first observation and a+t is the time of the second observation of the same attribute in the same observation unit). The frequency distributions are computed for several values of t and critical regions are defined, for which the probability α of the error first kind is given (Fig. 5.19). Because the dispersion of the interindividual random variable $Y = X^{(1)}-X^{(2)}$ for two randomly drawn different observation units (1) and (2) is greater than the dispersion of D_t, a larger part of Y is located in the critical region. Therefore, when results are misattributed, the probability β that this confusion is supposed will be greater than α. The greater the difference $\beta-\alpha$, the better an attribute is suited for detecting misattributed results.

An even greater certainty is obtained by simultaneous consideration of k attributes. The problem is reduced to the univariate case by introducing a **distance** function in the k-dimensional space.

5.2.2.2 Error Control in the Clinical Laboratory

In clinical laboratories there are explicit rules for error control, which (in Germany, at least) are partly set by law [121]. The types of control are distinguished as follows:

- **calibration control**, comprising the analysis of control sera with a known desired value, and
- **precision control**, comprising the analysis of control sera with an unknown desired value.

Furthermore, laboratories are obliged to take part in **Reference Sample** programs. These are usually cooperative programs where the same specimen is analyzed in different laboratories.

In **calibration control**, the standardized random variable

$$Y = \frac{X-\mu}{\sigma}$$

is computed from the result X, the desired value μ, and the standard deviation σ. However, the standard deviation σ is in general dependent on μ. Depending on the laboratory, an alarm is raised whenever the quotient exceeds a value of 2 or 3.

Precision control differs from calibration control only in that μ and σ are unknown and are estimated by the arithmetic mean $\bar{x}$ and the empirical standard deviation s of a series of determinations on the control serum itself. The results of subsequent tests are recorded on **control plots** over a time-axis, so that not only deviations from $\bar{x}$ but also trends can be recognized.

Additional determinations are performed on the control specimen throughout the day. Analyses of variance show that the day-to-day dispersion is usually about twice as large as the dispersion among repetitions on the same day, exhibiting the influence of the calibration and preparation of the control specimen.

5.2.2.3 Misspellings in Texts

Recognition and correction of misspellings is a semantic problem within medical linguistics (Chapter 4). The great importance of texts in medical information processing has raised the interest in simple, effective algorithms that can be employed in the control of large volumes of data, even if these algorithms cannot handle extremely difficult cases such as errors detectable only by semantic context analysis.

Recognition of misspellings can be simplified by reduction of the problem to the detection of formal errors in words, because then each admitted word can be listed in a dictionary. A word not found in such a list is either misspelled or is missing in the list and must be added.

The segmentation algorithms presented in Section 4.2.4 can also be employed for error control, because a misspelled word has a small probability of successful segmentation. The advantage of this approach is the smaller dictionary required; furthermore, the dictionary requires less frequent updating. On the other hand, these algorithms are intrinsically more complex.

Organization of automated detection of misspellings in texts depends on the organization of data acquisition (Section 5.2.1).

If the data are input at a terminal under program control, then the text can immediately be validated for misspellings, and necessary corrections can be made before any further data processing takes place. This reduces the overhead for corrections, which may sometimes burden routine work very much. If the domain is correspondingly reduced, then data input may even be done on micro-computers [138].

When texts are processed in batch-mode, for example, from OCR-forms, the possibility of manual corrections is lost. Because the texts are usually difficult and written under time-pressure, there is a significant incidence of misspellings. Therefore, in batch-mode error control should be complemented by methods for automated **error correction**. In order to do this, a misspelled word is replaced by that word from the dictionary that has the smallest distance. The distance functions cited in literature are frequently based on the HAMMING distance (Section 3.3.2.2.1.1). A comprehensive reference list and an algorithm is contained in [47], which can be implemented fairly easily and may correct the majority of misspellings occuring in routine texts.

Major problems arise in the control of misspellings in **names**. In many automated data files the name is part of the identification data (Section 5.1.3.7.1). The only control generally available, but a rather insecure one, is the control of letter sequences (**m-grams**), using the probability distribution of n-letter sequences in names. A sequence with a "small" probability indicates a misspelling.

5.2.2.4 Disturbance of Analog Messages

A **signal** Y(t) (Section 2.2.1) involves the **message** f(t) representing the information and the **disturbance** E(t) representing all errors:

$$Y(t) = f(t) + E(t) .$$

Disturbance is generated by the hardware (defect devices, improper application of sensors, variation of supply voltage) or by the individual (muscle potentials in EEG). The type of disturbance is systematic (inaccurate calibration, paroxysmal alterations in the ECG-signal) or asystematic (muscle potentials). In asystematic disturbances **noise** can be further distinguished from discrete disturbances.

The noise may be compared with the Brownian motion. It arises from the summation of many distinct and independent influences, all having expectation 0 and finite variance. Therefore, its distribution can be approximated by a $N(0, \sigma^2)$-distribution according to the central limit theorem [85].

The methods for extracting the message f(t) from the signal utilize **filters**. They can be classified as general methods or as specific methods, the latter ones being directed towards the nature of a specific error. Filters are better, when designed with knowledge of the source and frequency of the error. Specific filters are not presented here, because they are mathematically expensive [66]. But we illustrate the principles with a few examples (see also Section 6.1.2.1.1).

A **threshold** filter cuts off all values of Y(t) above (or below) a threshold λ, e.g.,

$$Y(t) \longleftarrow \min\Big(\lambda, Y(t)\Big) \quad , \qquad \text{or} \qquad Y(t) \longleftarrow \max\Big(\lambda, Y(t)\Big) .$$

A **band-pass** filter excludes all values of Y(t) outside a given range of t. A function is **smoothed** by an intervalwise approximation of Y(t), usually a polynomial function. Smoothing corresponds to the statistical method of **regression analysis**, where Y(t) is approximated stepwise (or as a whole) by a regression function (in the simplest case by a constant, e.g., the arithmetic mean).

The method of **sliding means** requires digitization of the data. The data y_i (i=1,2,...,n) are replaced by the mean computed from k neighbors:

$$y_i \leftarrow \frac{1}{k} \cdot \sum_{j=i}^{i+k-1} y_j \quad (i=1,2,\ldots,n-k+1) \; .$$

The marginal data $y_{n-k+2}, y_{n-k+3}, \ldots, y_n$ are usually omitted. Analogous to this "right" sliding means, "left" and "central" sliding means can be defined. In central sliding means, y_i is replaced by the mean:

$$y_i \leftarrow \frac{1}{k} \cdot \sum_{j=i-(k-1)/2}^{i+(k-1)/2} y_j \quad (i=(k+1)/2,\ldots,n-(k-1)/2), \quad k \text{ odd! } .$$

Computation of a **representative cycle** in periodic functions f(t) (e.g., ECG) is based on a statistical method. The limits t_i of the cycles are estimated in a first step. When the initial value t_0 is set to 0, λ_i is the length of a cycle, and λ is the mean length of all cycles, then

$$Y_i(t) = f(t) + E_i(t), \quad t_{i-1} \leq t \leq t_i \; (i=1,2,\ldots,n) \; .$$

The representative cycle is the mean function:

$$Y(t) \leftarrow \frac{1}{n} \cdot \sum_{i=1}^{n} Y_i\left(t_{i-1} + \frac{\lambda_i}{\lambda} \cdot t\right) \; , \; 0 \leq t \leq \lambda \; .$$

A filter is realized either in a program (software) or in a technical device (hardware). Software filters have the advantage of being more easily adjusted. Algorithms can be more rapidly developed, implemented, and modified, but they may use a considerable amount of processing time. If an algorithm is sufficiently simple and standardized, then it can be realized by electric circuits in an instrument. This realization is more expensive, but it speeds up processing time.

5.3 Data Storage

The logical data structure (Section 5.1.2) has to be distinguished conceptually from the physical data structure implemented on a specific storage medium. If the logical data structure is determined, then the physical data structure depends mainly on:

- storage type (internal storage, magnetic tape, magnetic disk, ...),
- operating system of the computer,
- programming language,
- efficiency considerations with respect to access mode (sequential, direct) and access frequency.

The reader is referred to [82] for detailed information about the different techniques.

5.4 Information Extraction

Information extraction comprises the methods for deriving values from input data for those attributes, which are specified by the model. Obviously, the first elementary step of information extraction is the creation of an object triplet. **Information integration** comprises the methods for relating object triplets by model-dependent relations to form informations on "higher" levels. Yet it is not worthwhile to distinguish these two concepts, because the recursive definition of an object triplet admits the explanation of "information integration" as "information extraction" (Section 5.1).

Information extraction is based on the storage and application of background knowledge (Section 5.1.2.3).

In PATIENT the data 210 mm Hg and 140 mm Hg are observed for the two attributes RR_{syst} (systolic blood pressure) and RR_{diast} (diastolic blood pressure), respectively. The first elementary step of information extraction is the formation of the two functions

$$\text{VALUE (PATIENT, } RR_{syst}) = 210 \quad \text{and} \quad \text{VALUE (PATIENT, } RR_{diast}) = 140$$

for the corresponding object triplets

$$\text{(PATIENT, } RR_{syst}, 210) \qquad \text{and} \quad \text{(PATIENT, } RR_{diast}, 140)\,.$$

From this information the information

$$\text{(PATIENT, } RR_{med}, 175)$$

can be deduced by averaging, i.e., employment of methodological knowledge (definition of the mean).

When medical knowledge is available, then further information can be deduced from elementary information. Thus, from the rule

IF VALUE (PATIENT, RR_{diast}) > 120 $\wedge$ VALUE (PATIENT, RR_{med}) > 150,
THEN VALUE (PATIENT, DIAGNOSIS) = 'renal or renovascular hypertension'

the new object triplet

(PATIENT, DIAGNOSIS, 'renal or renovascular hypertension')

is deduced by applying the rule to the data of PATIENT.

For additional examples of information extraction see Chapter 6.

5.4.1 Indexing

Indexing is the analysis and transformation of an utterance in medical language into elements of an utterance model (Chapter 4, Section 5.1.3.7). Components of the model are medical informations (Section 5.1.3.7.2) and their relations (Section 5.1.3.7.3). Because medical informations are denoted by lexemes, indexing and classification of concepts are closely associated.

Indexing may be compared with the processing of an ECG (Section 6.1.1.1). The ECG-curve contains most of the data. But information extraction, e.g., diagnosis, is impeded by a lack of knowledge relating details of the ECG to the diagnosis. In other words, the ECG-curve is redundant with respect to diagnosis.

In language utterances too, one is frequently interested only in a part of the information, which additionally may be classified.

If a surgeon is interested in the frequencies of complications of his operations, then the utterance "secondary infection after appendectomy in a 47 years old female patient with slight general reactions" contains excessive detail. The relevant information is contained in "secondary infection after appendectomy". If the type of complication is not required, then "secondary infection" has to be transformed into "complication".

Applications of indexing are found whenever language data have to be processed. Examples are computer-supported medical history taking (Section 5.1.3.5), diagnosis (Section 3.5.2.2), bibliography (Section 6.5), and documentation ("computerized medical record", Section 5.1.3.7.3; disease registers, Section 6.4).

Methods for automated indexing are necessary for several reasons:

- Manual indexing of massive amounts of data is very expensive and has a high error rate.
- There is a serious incompatibility between the qualification required of a human indexer and the monotony involved in indexing routine data.

5.4.1.1 Quality Measures

Quality of indexing can theoretically be described by the quality of the responses from a data base with indexed data:

A query divides the set S of utterances in the data base into a subset A of "relevant" utterances and the complementary set $\bar{A}$ of "irrelevant" utterances. We define B as the set of utterances in response to a query (Fig. 5.20).

Let the data base contain the indexed diagnoses for a set of patients. Then the query "retrieve all patients with appendicitis" divides the set of diagnoses into the set A of relevant diagnoses ('appendicitis', 'inflammation of vermiform appendix', 'inflammation of appendix vermiformis', ...) and the set $\bar{A}$ of irrelevant diagnoses.

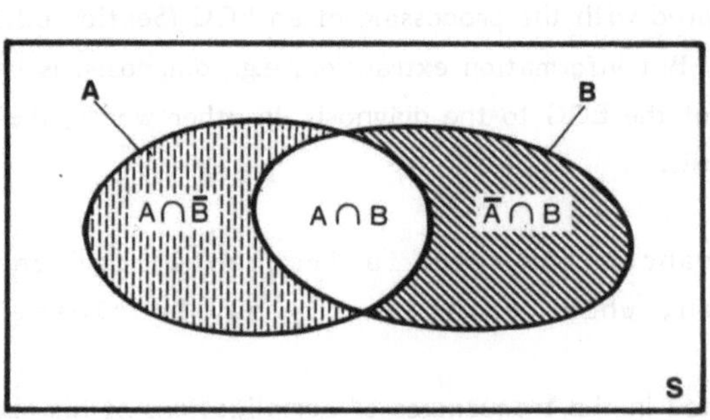

Fig. 5.20: VENN diagram for definition of quality measures in indexing. The set S of all utterances contains for a query a set A of relevant utterances. The set B of utterances is the response to the query

When d is an utterance contained in the data base, the response to a query may involve two types of errors:

(1) The relevant utterance d is not retrieved: $d \in (A \cap \bar{B})$.

(2) The irrelevant utterance d is retrieved: $d \in (\bar{A} \cap B)$.

These errors correspond to the following measures:

Recall $= P(d \in B | d \in A) = \dfrac{P(A \cap B)}{P(A)}$.

The response is more "complete", as more relevant utterances are retrieved (see "sensitivity" in Section 3.1.3).

Precision $= P(d \in A | d \in B) = \dfrac{P(A \cap B)}{P(B)}$.

The response is more "precise", as more utterances retrieved are relevant.

Often, these measures have only a theoretic meaning, because they can rarely be computed in practical applications. To compute these measures, the a priori-probabilities of all possible queries would have to be known, and for each possible query the sets A and B would have to be defined.

If the two measures are related to a specific query, then the a priori-probability is no longer needed, i.e., the probabilities in the definitions are replaced by the respective relative frequencies related to a special query. While the precision can now be estimated by analysis of the response, recall remains mostly unknown. In order to compute the recall, the data base would have to be divided into the sets A and $\bar{A}$ by some sort of an "outside criterion".

5.4.1.2 Methods

In a **descriptor-out-of-context** system the lexemes describing the text (**descriptors**) are added to the text; in a **descriptor-in-context** system the descriptors must be contained in the text.

A dictionary $\mathbf{L}$ containing the lexemes ℓ_i is given for indexing. The text t to be indexed may consist of words, $t = w_1 w_2 \ldots w_n$. In this section, character strings are interpreted as sets of words in order to avoid the introduction of an additional notation. The fact that a lexeme ℓ is a substring of t is, therefore, denoted by $\ell \subseteq t$; the fact that a word w is an element of t is denoted by $w \in t$.

We want to replace the text t by a set I of lexemes (**imdex**) such that the information content of t remains unchanged:

$$t \longleftarrow I = \{\ell_1, \ell_2, \ldots\} \;, \quad \ell_i \in L \;.$$

For example, different index levels for a book are title, content, and index.

5.4.1.2.1 Word-Oriented Methods

A simple approach is based on the postulation that each lexeme $\ell \in I$ must be a substring of t (descriptor-in-context): $\ell \subseteq t$.

When every lexeme is just a single word, this condition reduces to $\ell \in t$ and the dictionary becomes superfluous, because each text is represented by the set of all words. Such simple systems are offered by computer industry (STAIRS by the IBM Corporation, GOLEM/PASSAT by the SIEMENS AG). They have two serious disadvantages:

- In most applications the set of words is redundant. This results in excessive demand for storage capacity and in prolonged search times. In order to obtain a sufficient recall, the user must provide as many variations for his denotations as possible (Carcinom, Karcinom, Carzinom, Karzinom, ...).
- Information in idiomatic phrases is destroyed (dura mater).

Several techniques are employed in order to reduce redundancy:

- The dictionary is a **positive list** containing all words permitted for indexing (GOLEM/PASSAT).
- There is a **negative list** N containing all words not permitted for indexing. Usually, articles, pronouns, and expletives are elements of N. Then the indexing condition is

  $$\ell \in (t \cap \bar{N}) \;.$$

- The words of the text are transformed in order to represent synonyms by the same lexeme. Then the indexing condition is

  $$\ell \in \sigma(t) \;, \qquad \sigma(t) := \{\sigma_1(w_1), \sigma_2(w_2), \ldots\} \;.$$

Examples of such transformations are:

lemmatization	(corticale → cortical)
plural - singular	(hands → hand)
adjective - noun	(cortical → cortex)
synonym - preferred term	(kidney → ren) .

For example, lemmatization is incorporated into GOLEM/PASSAT. The same effect is reached in STAIRS by the ability to search not only on single words, but also on formally defined word sets. Thus, the key may be all words beginning with 'sick' with up to n additional characters (search key is 'sick$n').

Redundancy is further reduced by a dictionary of morphemes instead of words, relying on an algorithm utilizing that a phrase is not a random combination of words, a word is not a random combination of morphemes, and a morpheme is not a random combination of characters.

SNOP [183] contains 262,422 characters. However, when morphemes are coded, then SNOP contains only $14,340 \cdot 5.7 = 81,738$ morphemes. In addition, a morpheme dictionary is needed with $4,726 \cdot 4.9 \simeq 23,157$ characters (Table 5.5).

Unit	Number	Mean number of units per lexeme	Mean number of characters per unit
lexeme	14,340	1	18.3
word	11,116	2.1	10.4
morpheme	4,726	5.7	4.9

Table 5.5: Number of different lexemes, words, and morphemes in SNOP [183]

Two systems in medicine, which employ these techniques, are used for documentation in pathology [92,129,178]. The AGK-thesaurus [129,178] consists of two related word lists. Each word of the text must be contained in the list of about 70,000 "input words". Each input word is mapped explicitly on exactly one of the about 19,000 "standard words".

During the first step, each word of the text is replaced by its standard word (Fig. 5.21). This transformation comprises lemmatization, replacement of adjectives by nouns, replacement of synonyms by preferred words, and suppression of insignificant words (replacement by the null string). Therefore, the list of input words has the functions of a negative list as well as of a positive list.

In the second step, the standard words are classified according to six semantic dimensions and "associated" lexemes are supplied for compound words (references). In this step the "list" of standard words is utilized (Fig. 5.21, 5.22).

The same approach is employed to process queries. Any utterance qualifies for a query, when its set of descriptors contains the set of descriptors in the query. The supply of "associated" descriptors from the list of standard words corresponds to a descriptor-out-of-context system within a descriptor-in-context system.

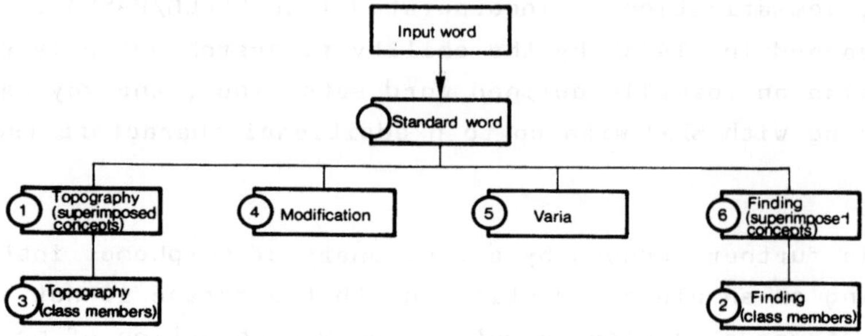

Fig. 5.21: Semantic structure of the AGK-thesaurus [129,178]. List of input words and list of standard words. Each standard word is assigned to one of six semantic dimensions and may be supplied with "associated" descriptors from these dimensions

Loss of information contained in idiomatic phrases can only be avoided when the dictionary $\mathbb{L}$ contains these phrases. Some word-oriented systems try to replace a phrase dictionary during processing the query. For example, multi-word phrases can be simulated by considering **neighborhood relations** (retrieve all utterances, containing the adjacent words "dura" and "mater"). For this type of search, the text replacement must include not only descriptors but also their position in the text.

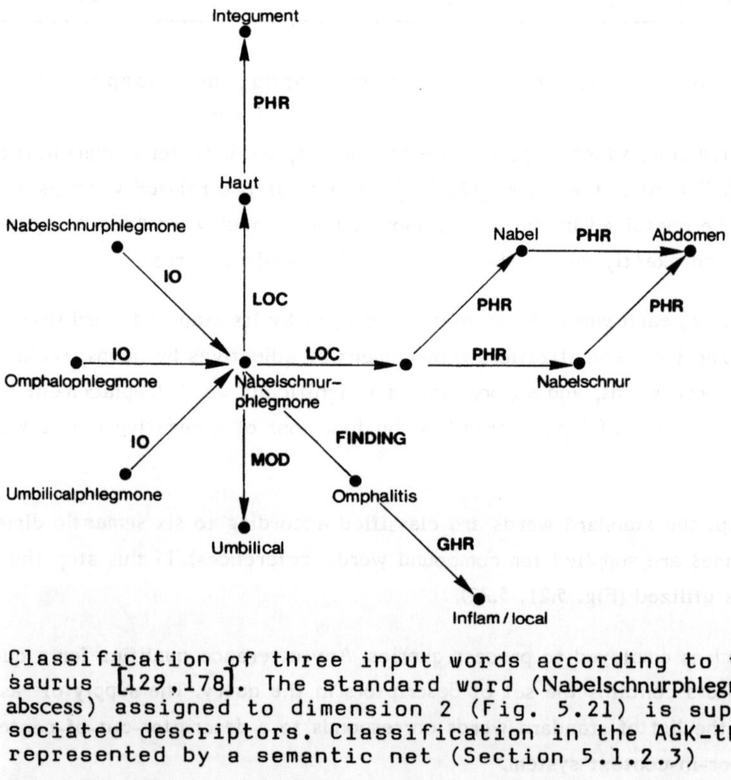

Fig. 5.22: Classification of three input words according to the AGK-thesaurus [129,178]. The standard word (Nabelschnurphlegmone ≙ navel abscess) assigned to dimension 2 (Fig. 5.21) is supplied by associated descriptors. Classification in the AGK-thesaurus is represented by a semantic net (Section 5.1.2.3)

5.4.1.2.2 Phrase-Oriented Methods

A phrase-oriented dictionary $\mathbb{L}$ is basically preferrable in order to improve precision. However, techniques have to be employed to avoid enormously increased redundancy in the dictionary.

Thus, the indexing condition $\ell \subseteq t$ for 'acute hemorrhagic inflammation' results in the index

$$\{\ell_1 = \text{'inflammation'}, \ell_2 = \text{'acute inflammation'}, \ell_3 = \text{'hemorrhagic inflammation'}\}.$$

But if the same statement can be formulated as 'inflammation, acute, hemorrhagic', then the dictionary must contain not only 'acute inflammation', but also lexemes such as 'inflammation, acute' in order to get a corresponding index.

Redundancy of such a dictionary is significantly reduced by substituting the equality as the indexing condition by the subset-relation between ℓ and t, and allowing transformation of the words (Section 5.4.1.2.1):

$$\ell \subseteq \sigma(t).$$

The above-described example points to a further possibility to reduce redundancy. The redundancy of ℓ_1 demonstrates that one lexeme must not be a (possibly transformable) substring of another lexeme in the same index:

$$\ell_i \subseteq \sigma(t) \quad (i=1,2,\ldots),$$

$$\ell_i \nsubseteq \ell_j \quad , \text{ for } i \neq j \; , \; \ell_i, \ell_j \in I \; .$$

This restriction corresponds to the **principle of longest match.** It is supported by the observation that for $\ell_i \subset \ell_j$ the lexeme ℓ_j often denotes a specialization of the concept denoted by ℓ_i or else ℓ_i is an artefact (for example, $\{\ell_1 = \text{'plasma'}, \ell_2 = \text{'plasma cell myeloma'}\}$).

However, this restriction is not generally valid.

'Inflammation, membraneous labyrinth' results in the index:

$$\{\ell_1 = \text{'inflammation'}, \ell_2 = \text{'inflammation, membraneous'}, \ell_3 = \text{'membraneous labyrinth'}\}.$$

From $\ell_1 \subset \ell_2$ and the condition $\ell_i \nsubseteq \ell_j$, the lexeme ℓ_1 would be suppressed. But the "correct" index is $\{\ell_1, \ell_3\}$.

Overlapping lexemes cannot be processed by general rules. A sufficient solution requires a combination of syntactic and semantic analysis (Section 4.3, 4.4).

The problem of indexing can also be formulated as follows:

An index I is a subset of lexemes ℓ_i from a dictionary $\mathbb{L}$, $I=\{\ell_1, \ell_2, \ldots\}$, with

$$\ell_i \subseteq \sigma(t),$$
$$\ell_i \nsubseteq \ell_j, \text{ for } i \neq j .$$

A **similarity function** f is defined on all permitted texts t and on all subsets $I \subset \mathbb{L}$ such that

$$f(t,I) \begin{cases} = 0, & \text{if I is not an index of t} \\ > 0, & \text{otherwise} \end{cases} .$$

An index I is a **best** index for a text t if $f(t,I) \geq f(t,J)$ for all subsets $J \subset \mathbb{L}$.

In practical medical applications by use of SNOMED [33] as the dictionary $\mathbb{L}$ the following approach has a demonstrated value:

(1) Overlapping of lexemes is excluded:

$$\ell_i \subseteq \sigma(t)$$
$$\ell_i \cap \ell_j = \epsilon \quad \text{for } i \neq j .$$

(2) Similarity of an index I with a text t increases, as

- the number s of morphemes of I increases
- the number m of lexemes of I decreases

} principle of longest match,

- the number u of words of t not contained in a lexeme ℓ_i (with all their morphemes) decreases

} syntactic restriction.

(3) Similarity is additive, i.e., if I_1 and I_2 are disjoint indexes of t, then

$$f(t, I_1 \cup I_2) = f(t, I_1) + f(t, I_2) \quad \text{for} \quad I_1 \cap I_2 = \{\epsilon\} .$$

From these three conditions the similarity function f is seen to be a linear function of s, m, and u, which has the following form after suitable normalization:

$$f(t, I) = a \cdot s - b \cdot m - u \quad , \; a, b > 0 \; .$$

In particular, it follows for an index containing a single morpheme as part of a word t:

$$a - b - 1 > 0 \quad \text{or} \quad a > b + 1 \; .$$

A system for automated processing of pathologic findings in medical language on the basis of SNOP [32] is described in [114,123,178]. It uses a whole set of sophisticated algorithms in order to cope with the irregularities of language and has demonstrated that the problem of automated indexing is basically solvable.

5.5 Information Retrieval

Information retrieval and presentation is the counterpart of data acquisition. Because an algorithm is largely influenced by the data to be processed and the results to be generated, the analysis of the "information needs" of a user is the center of systems analysis.

The primary results of laboratory data processing (Section 6.1.3) are object triplets. The obviously simplest form of information presentation is a table for each patient and day with the corresponding data. Thus, laboratory data processing makes an important contribution to the management of large amounts of data and makes transmission of data safer, faster, and partially cheaper than conventional methods. However, it is not at all certain that the receiving physician obtains better information (except for a decrease in error rate).

Technical preparation of a **table** exerts a strong influence upon interpretability. For example, closely related attributes (electrolytes, serum proteins) should be tabulated together. Temporal relationships among different attributes, or within the same attribute measured at different times in the same patient, should be considered in the arrangement. Much more complex is the field of decision support, for example, by automatically flagging abnormal values (Fig. 5.23).

Besides tabular representations, **graphic** representations are often very helpful.

Thus, the results of a standard test sequence with quantitative attributes (serum electrolytes) can be simultaneously represented in a circle diagram. Each attribute is assigned a radius. If the

B[redacted], A G N E S

INSTITUT F. KLINISCHE CHEMIE / LABOR-EDV
(BEFUND-AUSDRUCK AM 26.06.79 UM 15.59)

(7) 12A/1321

-1-

			W. NORMBEREICH	UHRZ'	17.06.79 SO	18.06.79 MO	19.06.79 DI	20.06.79 MI	21.06.79 DO	22.06.79 FR	23.06.79 SA
NATRIUM	(S)	MMOL/L	132 - 155		143	141	142	137	139	138	
KALIUM	(S)	MMOL/L	3,60 - 5,40		4,66	4,08	4,52	4,30	4,21	4,53	
CHLORID	(S)	MMOL/L	97 - 108			101	104	102	101	101	
PROTEIN	(S)	G/L	65 - 80			68	71		76		
CALCIUM	(S)	MMOL/L	2,15 - 2,75			2,16	2,29	2,12-	2,23	2,12-	
PHOSPHAT	(S)	MMOL/L	0,83 - 1,67			1,33	1,20	1,04	1,33	1,14	
GLUCOSE	(S)	MMOL/L	3,9 - 5,6			7,6+	7,7+		6,9+	6,4+	
HARNSTOFF	(S)	MMOL/L	3,3 - 6,7		16,0+	16,5+	14,6+		14,0+	11,3+	
KREATININ	(S)	UMOL/L	BIS 115		87	106	93	86	102	91	
GOT	(S)	U/L	BIS 15			8		16+			
GPT	(S)	U/L	BIS 17			17		15			
ALK.P'ASE	(S)	U/L	76 - 190			128		130			
GAMMA-GT	(S)	U/L	BIS 18			180+		151+			
CHE	(S)	U/L	1900 - 3800			1050-		1610-			
GLDH	(S)	U/L	BIS 3			2N		2N			
CHOLESTER.	(S)	MMOL/L	BIS 6,5	8'		4,8					
ALBUMIN	(S)	%	57 - 68	8'		47-					
ALPHA1-GL.	(S)	%	1 - 6	8'		6					
ALPHA2-GL.	(S)	%	5 - 11	8'		13+					
BETA-GL.	(S)	%	7 - 13	8'		11					
GAMMA-GL.	(S)	%	10 - 18	8'		23+					
KREAT.-CL.		ML/MIN	80 - 170			68-	72-	81	54-	52-	
KREAT.WAHR	(S)	UMOL/L	50 - 80			74	81+	91+	83+	90+	
KREATININ	(U)	MMOL/L				2,5	3,1K	3,9	2,7	3,2	
KREATININ	(U)	MMOL/D	9,0 - 14,0			7,3-	8,4-	10,5	6,5-	6,7-	
OSMOLALIT.	(S)	MOSM/KG	280 - 310	8'						302 /	
URINMENGE		ML				2900	2700	2700	2400	2100	
SAMMELDAUER		H				24	24	24	24	24	
PH	(U)		5 - 7			5	5	6	5		
PROTEIN	(U)					NEG.	+	NEG.	NEG.		
GLUCOSE	(U)					NEG.	NEG.	++	NEG.		
KETON-KOERPER	(U)					NEG.	NEG.	NEG.	NEG.		
HAEMOGLOBIN	(U)					NEG.	NEG.	NEG.	NEG.		
SEDIMENT	(U)					O.B.		O.B.	O.B.		
LEUKOZYTEN	(U)			7'			1-4				
ERYTHROZYTEN	(U)			7'			NEG.				

Fig. 5.23: Printing of the results of several analyses in the clinical laboratory of the Medical School Hannover for a female patient. Analyses have been performed between 6/17/1979 and 6/23/1979. The symbols indicate that a result is:

-: pathologically low
/: printed the first time
N: below the limit printed

+: pathologically high
K: verified by repetition of the analysis

The printing has been presented by Dr. A.J. PORTH

data are standardized for each attribute and the quotient is plotted on the corresponding radius, then "normal" results fall into a circular stripe around the unit circle. If the attributes are arranged in a clever order, then one gets characteristic deformations for certain diseases, i.e., a typical pattern (Fig. 5.24). The same information is much more difficult to extract from tables with several attributes.

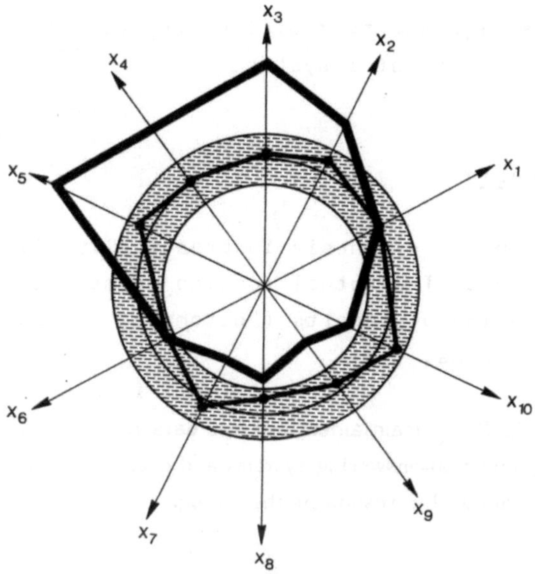

Fig. 5.24: Simultaneous representation of "normal" and "pathologic" standardized results of a test sequence with several quantitative attributes X_i. The "normal region" is hatched

The advantage of such representations of a disease as an easily recognizable and memorizable pattern may also be a reason for caution. On the one hand, the pattern depends strongly on the population, for which the results have been standardized. This leads to the problem of "normal" values already mentioned. On the other hand, such patterns are generated or hidden when the assignment of attributes to radiuses is changed. Therefore, the assignment should be chosen such that clear indications for important diseases or disease groups emerge. In order to reach this goal, correlated attributes have to be arranged on adjacent radiuses.

Time at which certain information is needed is another important point. The best data are useless if presented too late. Because the speed of information retrieval has a great influence on the costs of a computer system, a precise analysis of needs is necessary. It is comfortable and elegant to have all data directly accessible, but experience shows that this increases technical and financial costs, which only development projects can support. In other words, we must define for each application what **timely** presentation really means. Obviously, timeliness cannot be identical with **real-time**, i.e., direct data access.

Information retrieval and presentation is not only related to the technology of data processing and to medicine, but also to psychologic and social aspects of the users of a system.

5.5.1 Language Synthesis

The importance of language synthesis in practically all applications has already been pointed out. The actual domains in medicine are computer support in the generation of reports ("automated medical reporting") and question-answering systems.

This classification cannot rigidly be maintained, because data for automated medical reporting are frequently captured by question-answering systems and question-answering systems frequently generate a final report containing the results of the dialog.

5.5.1.1 Automated Medical Reporting

Development and employment of automated medical reporting is frequently initiated by the desire for labor saving. Medical reports are redundant on account of convention (Thank you for referring your patient ...), needs in human communication (error control), and demand for syntactically correct formulations.

An algorithm for the synthesis of a medical report has the following prerequisites:

- formal description of the structure of the medical report,
- availability of the data to be included in the medical report,
- rules for transformation of the internal codes of the data into the external representation to make the medical report readable for the recipient without additional information.

The need for a formal description derives from the prerequisite of a fixed internal and external structure of the medical report. The external structure is primarily defined by convention (e.g., position of address and reference). The internal structure depends on the relations among attributes and the criteria employed by the author.

The elementary unit is the object triplet (Section 5.1). In general, the relation between observation unit and attribute is represented by caption or textual arrangement (block, paragraph), and the relation between attribute and value is represented by caption or by local formatting, if the attribute cannot directly be derived from the denotation of the data.

The structure and the required transformations can be described by means developed for the description of formal languages.

A medical report (Fig. 5.25) may comprise location and calendar date (W), address (A), and text (T). The text involves reference (Betr.), salutation (An), introduction (Einl), admission findings (Abef), examinations (Unt), therapy (Th), final diagnoses (Dia), and termination (Schl). The sections can be further divided. Therefore, the syntax of the medical report Z is:

Z → W A T
W → 'Münster,' func3
A → Anr($S) β
T → Betr. An Einl Abef Unt Th Dia Schl
Betr. → 'Betr.:' Anr($S1) γ ', geb.' δ
An → 'Sehr' X1($S) Anr($S) X2($S)
Einl → 'Haben Sie vielen Dank für die Überweisung' X3($S1) X4($S1)
...
Dia → 'Abschließende Diagnosen:' D
D → func4($Y)
Anr → func2('Frau', 'Herr')
X1 → func2('geehrte', 'geehrter')
$S → func1(S)
S → 'F' | 'M'
X2 → func2('Kollegin!', 'Kollege!')
$S1 → func1(S1)
S1 → 'F' | 'M'
...

In this notation, constant character strings are enclosed in apostrophes and attribute names are denoted by lower case Greek letters, which are replaced by the corresponding external data representation in the written medical report. Symbols beginning with a $ are also attribute names, but have an additional meaning. Thus, in Anr($S) the argument $S is replaced by the consecutive number of the value of S, equal to the corresponding datum (value of the function func1).

The function func2 selects from a list the element corresponding to this number and substitutes this element in the text. For example, if the datum of the attribute S is 'M', then $S results in 2 and Anr(2) results in 'Herr'. The function func3 substitutes the calendar date. The function

```
                                          Münster, 10.3.1979

Frau
Dr. Erna Arzt
---
Betr.: Frau A. Müller, geb. 12.7.23

Sehr geehrte Frau Kollegin!

Haben Sie vielen Dank für die Überweisung Ihrer Patientin A. Müller.
Die Patientin wurde in unserer Klinik vom 26.2.1979 bis zum 6.3.1979
stationär behandelt. Bei der stationären Aufnahme bestand ein Ver-
dacht auf Diabetes mellitus.

Die körperliche Untersuchung ergab:
           Blutdruck: 190/110 (im Stehen)
           ---

Es wurden folgende Laboruntersuchungen vorgenommen:
           Nüchternblutzucker: 230 mg/100 ml
           ---

Ergebnisse weiterer Untersuchungen:
           Augenhintergrund: Gefäße: ...
                             ---
         ---

Die Patientin wurde auf folgende Therapie eingestellt:
         ---

Abschließende Diagnosen:
           Diabetes mellitus
           Essentielle Hypertonie

                                  Mit kollegialen Grüßen
```

Fig. 5.25: Schema of an automatically generated medical report

func4 has the same task as func1, but includes a repetition instruction ("repeat for each value of the attribute Y").

The example shows that at least two classes of functions are required: a class for general tasks independent of the type of medical report (e.g., substitution of the calendar date, selection from a list) and a class dependent on the special type of medical report.

The second sentence of the letter applies only for inpatients. Therefore, a function is required, which determines whether the datum corresponding to the attribute "admission" is "inpatient" or "outpatient", before this part of the medical report is generated.

Besides the functions already mentioned, the formal description also includes rules for transformation of the codes (e.g., the transformation of S='M' into 'Herr').

Semantic functions form an important class, based on principles that can only be illustrated here, because this most complex part needs further development before it can be systematically presented.

Let "inflammation" be the datum of the attribute "morphology", and "lung, right" and "lung, left" be the data of the attribute "topography". A simple formal approach, employing only the relation between morphology and topography, results in the formulation "inflammation, lung, right; inflammation, lung, left". In order to get the medically more "elegant" formulation "bilateral pneumonia", two semantic transformations have to be made, one utilizing that "pneumonia" is the denotation of an inflammation in the lung, the other utilizing that the lung is a bilateral organ.

The costs of automated medical reporting depend mainly on structure and volume of the report. In general, a compromise between efforts for data acquisition and complexity of the algorithm has to be found.

In the above example, the medical report could also formally be defined by a single production:

$$Z \longrightarrow \alpha.$$

In other words, the medical report consists of the value of a single compound attribute fully formatted to the algorithm. Then the algorithm functions like a typewriter. This form is frequently used, when the medical report is the primary data source for a storage and retrieval system.

Between this extreme and the complete generation of the medical report from object triplets for primitive attributes, a whole set of transitions may be realized. An example is programmed text processing, in which parts of a text are inserted into a schema stored on a magnetic device. This approach does not pertain to language synthesis in the strict sense.

If the data needed for a medical report have already been acquired, for example, in the setting of fundamental documentation, then implementation will cause no serious problems [102]. The situation is more complex when the formal structure of the medical report presents the basis of a question-answering system for the acquisition of the required data [83]. Even in very sophisticated systems this leads to many difficulties; some systems have failed in daily use even after intensive and well-motivated development efforts.

In [184], automated medical reporting is described as a by-product of data acquisition for indexing. In addition, the data are utilized in the editing of several journals. Medical report systems in radiology are described in [84,100] that permit modifications and additions formulated in medical language in order to keep the relatively rigid schema from becoming too complex and to decrease the number of attribute levels.

5.5.1.2 Question-Answering Systems

Question-answering systems in medical applications can be found in:

- computer-supported medical history taking (Section 5.1.3.5),
- computer-aided instruction (CAI),
- consultant systems (Section 3.5.2.2),
- computer-supported acquisition of findings.

Most developments in these areas do not employ true language synthesis for communication but purely technical means:

The user has to present answers to fixed questions, selected from a fixed set of answers and presented on a terminal together with the questions (multiple-choice, menu-technique).

Such systems are rapidly and easily developed. They are widely applicable for textual input and require simple algorithms. Consequently, many have been published. Their main disadvantage is the rigid structure, which relies on a predefined explicit network, efficient in practice, but difficult to alter when relations are altered (Section 5.1.3.5). These algorithms are essentially independent of the specific application.

Systems employing models capable of properly representing facts, relations, and reasoning are significantly better in human interactive dialog. Although great advances have been made in the last few years [27], we are still far from a demonstrated "intelligent" dialog system, at least by the criterion of [161]: that a user cannot decide whether his partner is a computer system or a human by the dialog questions and answers. The problems to be solved can be arranged in five areas [26] (Section 5.1.2.3):

(1) **Representation of knowledge.**

(2) **Triggering of deductions**: Under what conditions are deductions made (immediately when new knowledge is captured, or later when a deduction is needed)?

(3) **Organization**: How are the elements of knowledge organized in order to find the knowledge required for reasoning?

(4) **Technique of deducing knowledge**: How are the elements of knowledge employed in reasoning?

(5) **Background**: What knowledge about the world enables humans to understand language?

5.6 Data Integrity

The data stored in an information system need to be protected with respect to the **state** of the data base and with respect to **access** to the data base. A data base may become incorrect when either false data are acquired or programs, processing, or technical devices are in error. The resulting loss of **data consistency** has to be distinguished from **data protection**. For special data protection problems in medical applications, resulting from legal requirements concerning confidential medical communication, the reader is referred to [57,79].

5.6.1 Data Consistency

The problems arising from the acquisition of false data have been discussed in Section 5.2.2. Errors in programs should be avoided by suitable means during program development and testing (Section 2.2.9), but there is no absolute safety in complex algorithms.

Basically, **consistency conditions** for a data base may be formulated in the application programs as well as in the definition of the data base by means of the data description language (DDL). The more sophisticated DDL's may relieve the application programs from much of the consistency checking (Section 5.1.1).

The DDL may provide data checks with respect to a definite set of permitted values (Section 5.2.2.1.1). Frequently, the data manipulation language provides additional data checks to ensure data integrity. Thus, in a hierarchic model (Section 5.1.1.2) special access paths have to be utilized for deletion or update of nodes.

Critical situations arise for every data base when either operations consist of sequential alterations or, as is usually the case, several users make changes simultaneously. The mechanisms related to these situations are summarized by **process integrity**.

A data base containing admission number ADMNO, NAME, and WARD for inpatients may be realized by two relations (Section 5.1.1.1):

ADMNO	NAME
00001/79	NAME1
00002/79	NAME2
---	---

ADMNO	WARD
00001/79	3A
00002/79	4
---	---

Then, both tables must be updated at a patient admission. But if updates are performed sequentially, the data base is then necessarily inconsistent after the first update. Any interruption of processing at this moment may allow the inconsistency to persist.

Simultaneous updating of the data base by several users has special requirements in order to make sure that alterations do not get lost.

A data base may contain a table for a compound object including admission number ADMNO, admission date ADMDAT, discharge date DSCHDAT, and discharge diagnosis DSCHDIAG:

ADMNO	ADMDAT	DSCHDAT	DSCHDIAG

Discharge date may be inserted by the administrative unit. At the "same" time discharge diagnosis may be inserted by the physician. In order to alter the data base, the application program must read the respective node into main storage and must restore the updated node. Then the following process leads to the loss of the discharge diagnosis:

Operation	State of the data base			
Update program for discharge diagnosis reads the data; Update program for discharge date reads the same data	00057/79	2.4.79		
Update program for discharge diagnosis writes the updated data back	00057/79	2.4.79		'APPENDICITIS'
Update program for discharge date writes the updated data back	00057/79	2.4.79	10.4.79	

This situation appears always when several updates of the same element in the data base overlap. It could be avoided by enforcing a strict time sequence upon alterations. But the system must allow overlapping of update processes, because only then is a large data base available to many users. The way out is to inhibit access by any other user to just those data to be altered, until the update is completed. The set of data to be blocked depends on the set of data which a process is updating, on the data model, and on the data base schema [98].

Data security comprises the precautions taken to protect data against loss or damage and procedures for restoring a data base after such an incident. It should be kept in mind that consequential loss from damage to a data-relation may exceed the direct loss by far (for example, the consequences of the loss of a patient identification in a data base keyed by this datum).

Loss or damage of data may be caused by errors in programs, system failures, or technical defects.

Data backup at regular intervals is the most frequent precaution. For example, the total data base may be copied onto magnetic tapes. Alterations performed between two copies may additionally be recorded on update tapes (log-tapes). When the data base is lost, then the copy is recopied and the intermediate alterations are repeated by special programs.

Frequency and time of data backup depend primarily on update frequency, costs of damages, and operational organization, because the entire data base is blocked during backup procedures.

5.6.2 Data Protection

Prevention of unauthorized access to the data base differs from the security measures described in the preceding section, in that access protection relates to communication lines, programs, and data. In recent years many countries have enacted special laws governing unauthorized access.

Protection against unauthorized access to **communication lines** comprises both controlling physical and electronic access to terminals.

Access to **programs** and **data** is usually controlled by checking a user identification. The user has to identify himself by a **password**; the system determines by a table search whether or not he is permitted to use the demanded program.

The selective protection of access to data is more difficult to realize and easier to penetrate. Basically, it can be realized by a permission matrix, the rows of which are assigned to users and the columns are assigned to attributes.

The costs, degree of safety, and obstruction of access in data protection systems are all interrelated and will have to be optimized for each individual application.

The importance of user cooperation is illustrated by an incident where the security of a very clever data protection scheme was broken, because an authorized user left his password on a piece of paper beside a terminal in a room accessible to every member of the hospital without any supervision.

A serious problem arises in attempting to control application programs. A program cannot be allowed to access the data base until it has been certified as correctly accessing only authorized data. Thus, it is possible to exclude the unauthorized access of programmers to the data base.

6. Special Applications

In this chapter, a brief overview of special computer-oriented or computer-supported applications is presented, without discussing implementation details of purely local interest.

6.1 Processing of Process Data

6.1.1 Biosignal Processing

Biosignals are primarily electric potentials resulting from biologic activities (e.g., ECG, EEG, EMG, ERG). Processing is frequently partitioned into **preprocessing** and actual **analysis**. In general, preprocessing includes transduction, amplification, analog-digital conversion (A/D-conversion, Section 2.2.3), and filtering (Section 5.2.2.4).

Algorithms used to analyze biologic functions represented in biosignals are mathematically very expensive. Their use is only worthwhile if reliable data are guaranteed by standardized careful recording techniques. Standards for ECG-recording and for the necessary equipment have been developed [87,120].

There are many interesting clinical applications of biosignal processing to diagnosis of diseases of the

- heart (ECG, intracardial pressure, phonocardiograms [41]),
- lungs (pulmonary function tests),
- muscles or nerves (EMG),
- eye (ERG),
- central nervous system (EEG).

6.1.1.1 Electrocardiography

Automated ECG-analysis has been developed to the point that it can be employed in routine clinical practice [112,119,193]. Tests have shown that modern computer-supported ECG-analysis programs, as they are commercially available, are superior to cardiologists in some diagnostic situations.

Analysis includes the twelve **standard leads** and/or the three **orthogonal leads** (vectorcardiography, VCG). Most authorities agree that both groups of leads contain the same amount of clinical information. VCG has the advantage of a significantly smaller intraindividual variation, but is usually combined with standard leads, for which more clinical experience is available.

The typical course of an ECG-analysis is:

- **Data acquisition**: Acquisition of the patients identification data and of additional data that depend on the evaluation program (differential diagnoses, medication, age, sex, ...). The ECG is either recorded on magnetic tape for later analysis (offline) or directly input (online) to the computer and analyzed in real time.
- **Preprocessing**: Data are digitized, filtered (Section 5.2.2.4), and any trend in the base line (isoelectric line) is corrected. The cycles are located and a representative cycle is determined and measured (P-, Q-, R-, S-, T-wave, ST-segment, see Fig. 2.6 in Section 2.2.3.1).
- **Classification**: Diagnostic evaluation based on the measured attributes.

In VCG the spatial and temporal alterations of a 3-dimensional vector are determined from its components given by the three X,Y,Z leads. Thus, P-wave, QRS-complex, and T-wave are determined by characteristic changes in the spatial speed V(t):

$$V(t) = \sqrt{\left(\frac{dX}{dt}\right)^2 + \left(\frac{dY}{dt}\right)^2 + \left(\frac{dZ}{dt}\right)^2} \quad .$$

Classification algorithms have a greater variability. Individual variations in approach differ so much that most ECG-systems provide diagnostic criteria that may be adapted to the individual user. For a survey of the most common codes the reader is referred to [105].

Problems in ECG-diagnosis arise, because findings vary for the "same" disease and are interpreted differently by different cardiologists.

Both problem groups are approached in modern ECG-analysis by multivariate statistical methods. Based on verified findings in a "training sample" (e.g., by autopsy) several hundred parameters are reduced to about 10 to 20 (Section 3.3). These parameters are assigned weights computed from the "training sample" such that as many cases as possible are correctly classified. Subsequently, these weights are used for classification of an unknown ECG ("test sample").

Variations of the previously described ECG-analysis are available for special situations, among which **rhythm analysis** is clinically most important. Special programs consider the methodological problems in the analysis of arrhythmic ECGs. An important clinical application is the surveillance of patients in intensive-care medicine (Section 6.1.5).

Other applications that make use of classification algorithms are intrauterine diagnosis and monitoring the fetus during labor [90].

Automated ECG-analysis offers the possibility of maintaining a large data base, which, for its part, can be utilized to improve analysis. An ECG-analysis system is cheaper than manual evaluation if it is utilized intensively. Furthermore, it is independent of the availability of clinical experts. Thus, several ECG-analysis systems accept telephone input and return the evaluation on the same line.

6.1.1.2 Electroencephalography

Progress in automated EEG-analysis has been significantly slower than for ECG, primarily, because the theory of EEG-signals and their most important parameters is inadequate [77]. Costly mathematical methods are required. These include computation of auto- and cross-correlation for detection of (missing) periodicities of rhythm, frequency analyses such as FOURIER analysis, and frequency spectra. Further investigation is needed of EEG-alterations evoked by specific stimuli (evoked potentials).

Determination of **evoked potentials** is based on the same principle as determination of a representative cycle (Section 5.2.2.4). A stimulus (e.g., light) is given at defined times t_i, evoking a response in the EEG in the interval $t_i \leq t \leq t_i + \lambda$. But the signal/noise ratio is usually too small for a valid interpretation. However, by periodic repetition of the stimulus, the ground activity in the EEG is overlaid with a periodic response. If the signal is then processed as a periodic function, then the responses to the stimuli accumulate in the representative cycle, while the ground activity is smoothed as it approximates a random signal, thus improving the signal/noise ratio.

6.1.2 Image Processing

Many applications such as smears (blood count, PAPANICOLAOU smears), X-ray images, ultrasonic "images", chromosome images, and scintigrams require the evaluation of 2-dimensional images.

Some important reasons for the great interest of medicine in automated image processing are:

- large volume of examinations with high costs in personnel and time (e.g., smears),
- unreliability of routine tests ("estimation" of the number of basophile or eosinophile leukocytes from a sample of 100 cells),
- replacement of dangerous or highly troubling examinations with non-invasive procedures (e.g., use of computer tomography rather than encephalography or multiple X-ray tomograms).

Many problems arise in automated image processing. Often the development of special instruments is necessary (e.g., automatic microscope for processing blood counts).

The amount of primary data for image analysis is very large. A black-and-white image is partitioned into individual points (like a newspaper picture), and each point is completely described by its two coordinates in the picture plane and its intensity (grey level). For sufficient resolution the distance between points must be small. Operations on the data are relatively simple, but the large amount of points burdens even large computers. For this reason, special computers are developed to carry out these operations simultaneously for a set of points.

The multiplicity of algorithms for image processing has become so great, and the algorithms have become so complex that specific knowledge is necessary to understand them. A complete overview would go far beyond the scope of this book [66,125].

6.1.2.1 Algorithms

Objectives of automated image processing include:

- contrast enhancement between **background** and **objects**,
- filtering,
- arithmetic and logical operations on images,
- geometric operations on images (translation, rotation, magnification),
- morphologic analysis, separation and localization of objects,
- classification.

6.1.2.1.1 Contrast Enhancement

Improvement of the image quality is an important prerequisite of image analysis. The simplest method for **contrast enhancement** is the use of threshold value filters. Usually, the threshold value is set by the user, but there are algorithms, which determine this information from the image itself.

Spatial filters for smoothing the image are more complex. Thus, isolated artifacts may be levelled out. These methods are employed for the detection of margins, edges, and finally "forms" in an image.

Assume an image section consisting of points with coordinates (x_i, y_i) and intensity z_i. Let intensity be a non-negative integer. In Fig. 6.1 a schema for values of the intensities of an approximately "ideal" bright line at x=3 is represented. Because of line-broadening and disturbances, intensity differs from 0 on both sides of x=3.

The most important contrast enhancement algorithms for analog data are based on differentiation and for digital data on differencing. Fig. 6.1 contains the results for the (left) difference:

$$f(x_i, y_i) \leftarrow \left| f(x_{i+1}, y_i) - f(x_i, y_i) \right| .$$

Improvements are often made by use of the second-order difference (Fig. 6.1):

$$f(x_i, y_i) \leftarrow \left| f(x_{i+1}, y_i) - 2 \cdot f(x_i, y_i) + f(x_{i-1}, y_i) \right| .$$

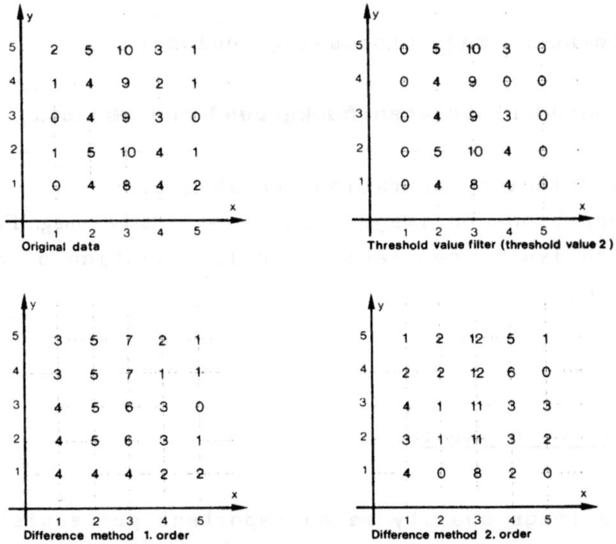

Fig. 6.1: Intensity of an image section and results of several methods for contrast enhancement. Intensity at the margins of the image is assumed to be 0

The operation performed in the x-direction is usually performed in both directions (spatial filtering). The generalization of the first-order differential is:

$$f(x,y) \leftarrow \sqrt{\left(\frac{\delta f}{\delta x}\right)^2 + \left(\frac{\delta f}{\delta y}\right)^2} \; .$$

The generalization of the second-order differential is the LAPLACE operator:

$$f(x,y) \leftarrow \left| \frac{\delta^2 f}{\delta x^2} + \frac{\delta^2 f}{\delta y^2} \right| \; .$$

Because these methods may not only enhance the contrast, but also increase the noise, they are frequently combined with smoothing techniques. A popular spatial smoothing method fits a second-degree polynomial to the data.

These methods are also used iteratively. For further information the reader is referred to [127,134,135,136].

These methods are modified for binary images, i.e., images with intensity 0 or 1. Binary images are generated by the application of "statistical tests":

> Let H_0 be the null hypothesis. For each point H_0 is tested. If H_0 is rejected, then the point is assigned the value 0; otherwise it is assigned the value 1.

6.1.2.1.2 Arithmetic Operations

The most important arithmetic operations are addition and subtraction of images after centering. Image subtraction has several applications such as:

- investigation of time-dependent processes (intake/elimination of radionuclides, growth tendencies of tumors),
- selective representation of isotope intake in certain organs. For example, the isotopes stored in the pancreas are also stored in the liver, which partially overlaps the pancreas. Subtraction of the liver image from the total image provides a representation of the pancreas intake.

Addition of images may improve signal/noise ratio, as in the determination of a representative cycle (Section 5.2.2.4).

6.1.2.1.3 Image Analysis

Algorithms for image analysis are not presented here, because they are sometimes very special and complex. Morphologic analyses (edge detection, localization and measuring of objects) are relatively simple in contrast to classification algorithms, which are similar in many ways to linguistic algorithms (Chapter 4).

In practical applications such as analysis of X-ray images [99], interactive input has a demonstrated value. A human expert takes over that share, which he can do particularly well (selection of interesting image sections and structures) and the computer takes over that share, which can well enough be defined by algorithms (contrast enhancement, application of statistical tests).

6.1.2.2 Computer-Tomography

Computer-tomography contrasts sharply with computer-supported image analysis. Hardly any other application area of mathematical or computer-supported methods in patient care has received such wide attention.

The "classical" X-ray picture is produced by passing a beam of X-rays through the body to a photographic film located at the opposite side. The beam is partially absorbed and dispersed depending on the density, thickness, and composition of the intervening structures, producing a shadow photograph of the irradiated body. The shadowgraph has two deficiencies:

- The minimum differences that the human eye can recognize in size and intensity amounts to some 5%. In practice, therefore, the radiologist can frequently differentiate only adipose tissues and structures containing gas, water, calcium, or heavy metals.

  Contrast can be enhanced by substances, which absorbe irradiation (barium or iodine compounds), or by filling cavities with air.

- The shadowgraph projects a 3-dimensional structure onto a 2-dimensional plane. The resulting superposition of structures blurs actual contrasts.

  In certain applications, these deficiencies are remedied by **tomography**. In this technique, X-ray beam and film are moved in coordination such that the points of one layer are mapped onto the same image points, whereas points from other layers are mapped onto different image points. This results in a clearer definition of the interesting layer while simultaneously blurring structures from other layers. The signal/noise ratio of such an image and the gradual transition to the interesting layer may cause serious difficulties in interpretation.

Computer-tomography (**CT**) essentially applies mathematical methods to **reconstruct** the tomographic image. The X-ray beam penetrating the body is projected onto a **detector** instead of a film and intensity is converted to digital values at each point and input to a computer (Fig. 6.2).

An algorithm constructs an image of the interesting layer from many points from the position/intensity values [126]. The interesting layer is beamed from different angles, and the algorithm eliminates the effects of superposition by considering the angle and the physical characteristics of the different tissue components (e.g., absorption coefficients of air and water). Some algorithms may transform intensity levels or absorption levels into different colors for enhanced contrast. The image may be displayed on a color monitor.

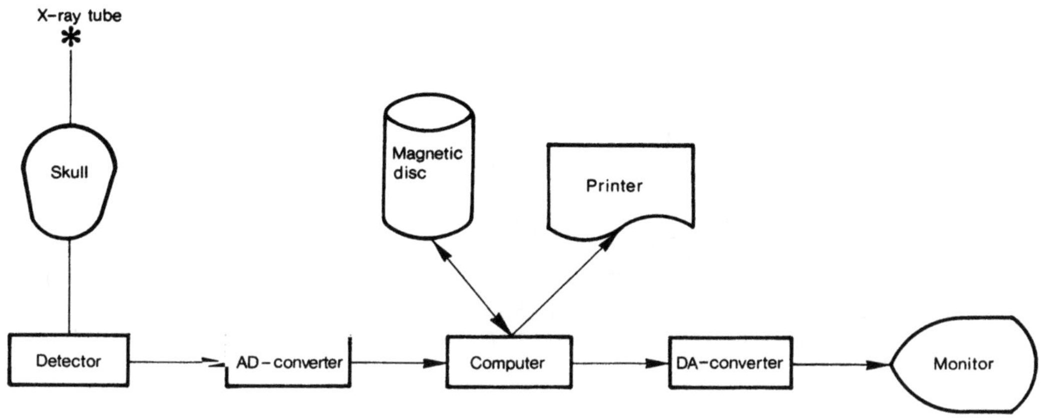

Fig. 6.2: Schema of a computer-tomograph

The most important advantage of computer-tomography is the higher resolution of optical density. Consequently, there is an enhanced definition and contrast of structures, showing features, which could previously be recognized only at autopsy.

Computer-tomography has developed in four "generations":

- The first generation comprises an X-ray tube and a single diametrically opposed detector. After each measurement, the system is moved along a measuring line (translation) and is rotated by 1°. This motion is repeated in a semicircle (**scanning**). The procedure takes a great deal of time (up to 5 minutes) and can, therefore, be applied only for examining fixed structures (e.g., skull).
- In the second generation, the number of detectors is increased up to 30 so that the translation step can be increased, thereby decreasing examination time to about 20 seconds.
- In the third generation, the number of detectors is further increased and the detectors are arranged in a segment of a circle. Thus, translation can be totally omitted. The system rotates around the longitudinal axis of the examinated body. Examination time is reduced to a few seconds.
- In the fourth generation, the detectors are arranged in a full circle and the X-ray tube rotates in this circle (Fig. 6.3).

The medical significance of these developments so far has been demonstrated in some areas. In other areas it can only be suggested; research is still going on and technologic development has partially advanced faster than clinical applications, some of which include:

- improvement of diagnosis (brain tumors, differential diagnosis of "stroke"),
- improvement of therapy (dosage planning for tumors because of more precise localization, testing of responses to therapy),
- replacement of dangerous or troubling methods (craniotomy, pneumencephalography, cerebral angiography).

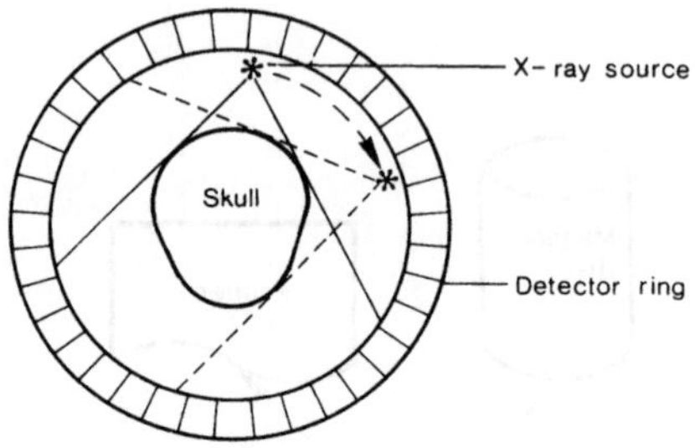

Fig. 6.3: Schema of a computer-tomograph of fourth generation. The irradiation source (*) rotates inside the detector circle around the object

A further important advance occurs in **emitting scanners**, where the interesting structure itself becomes the radiation source by application of radioactive substances. The medical consequences of the possible quantitative investigation of body functions and metabolic processes can now hardly be overlooked, as in the determination of

- cerebral activities by radioactively labelled glucose compounds (diagnosis of circulation problems),
- activity of tumors by measuring RNA formation and its factors (effects of treatment).

6.1.3 Laboratory Data Processing

Development of comprehensive and useful computer-based systems in the laboratory has reached a level of utility, which is higher than in most other areas of a hospital. This results from the high degree of automation, the repetitive nature of the work, the greater receptiveness to computer support, and the shortage of qualified personnel. "Turn-key"-systems are already offered by industry. The development of automated laboratory data processing has taken over tasks to be done elsewhere within the hospital environment (Section 6.3).

A rough classification of laboratory data processing includes the following subsystems:

- test requests,
- specimen distribution,
- data acquisition and input,
- data control and evaluation,
- data transmission.

There are four interfaces with the "environment" of the laboratory:

(1) **Test requests** coming from wards or ambulatory units have to be acquired, input, and

(2) linked to a **master data** file (medical record number, name, sex, age,...). Linkage to the master data file is needed for identification, medical control ("normal" values), and administration (billing).

(3) **Data** generated in the laboratory have to be transmitted to the requesting station and

(4) **administration** has to receive data relevant for billing.

Test requests and master data are usually hand-written on request sheets and are acquired into the laboratory computer in a secondary process. Test results are printed in the laboratory and transmitted with the normal internal mail to the requesting station (Fig. 5.23 in Section 5.5).

The best-known laboratory data processing systems in Germany are operated in the Medical School Hannover [121], at the hospital München-Harlaching [80,81], and at the University of Tübingen [103].

6.1.4 Radiology, Nuclear Medicine

Computer applications in radiology and nuclear medicine are found in diagnostic procedures, therapy, and documentation [185]. In **diagnostic procedures**, particularly in nuclear medicine, automated image processing has an important role (Section 6.1.2).

While automated analysis of X-ray images still requires additional research and development, industry offers "turn-key"-systems, for example, for evaluating scintigrams and for documenting the results (Section 6.1.2.2).

In **therapy**, programs for dosage planning have become of great interest. The objective is to plan the irradiation of a tumor (irradiation field, -angle, -duration, -intensity) so that an effective dose is given while minimizing iritation of normal tissue. Such programs are already available for use on desk-top calculators (for references see [38]).

In **documentation**, radiology reports contain a relatively high content of standard phraseology, and these reports can easily be structured. Consequently, automated reporting has been frequently described (Section 5.5.1.1).

6.1.5 Intensive-Care Medicine

The degree of mechanization in this subfield of clinical medicine is already so advanced that computer support can be considered to be a necessity. It would, however, be false to assume that computer-supported patient surveillance is merely data processing applied to a human message source.

Therapy based on the results of **intensive-care monitoring** requires the observation of qualitative and quantitative attributes and the evaluation of data utilizing medical knowledge. Qualitative attributes include color of skin, degree of consciousness, and responsiveness, while quantitative attributes include arterial and venous blood pressure, cardiac rhythm, respiratory rhythm, excretion of fluids, and biosignals. These data vary in time, and their relations to the "state" of a patient are not operationally defined. In no other subfield of medicine diminishes the importance of stating a "classical" diagnosis more with respect to treatment. The indispensable requirements of reliability, availability, and fast and safe action makes intensive-care medicine the application area, which is most sensitive to computerized procedures.

Biosignal processing has already been developed to the point of supplying medical and paramedical personnel with additional and reliable data (Section 6.1.1).

The intrinsic objective of early recognition of life-threatening trends and indications for intervention has not yet been reached [89,157]. Technical problems are partly responsible for this situation (development of proper sensors for signal acquisition, preprocessing of data, transmission of data), however, semantic problems are even more difficult. Intensive-care medicine has demonstrated that the efforts to develop algorithms are the most important means to clearly defining the problems, an essential step in their resolution.

6.2 Economic Applications

There is a broad spectrum of economic applications in medicine, because hospitals are large-scale economic enterprises. With few exceptions, these applications relate to medical informatics, because there is hardly any datum, which is of interest only to hospital administration.

The most important applications are:

- patient pre-admission scheduling,
- patient admission (including transfer and discharge),
- accounting,
- billing,
- menu-planning and food-distribution,
- inventory systems.

Among these applications we present only patient admission (because of its central role) and inventory systems (because of their algorithmic problems).

6.2.1 Patient Admission

Except for pre-admission appointments, patient admission marks the first contact of a patient with the hospital. It is an administrative procedure, which includes collecting demographic data and signing treatment-consent forms. As long as the data, obtained during patient admission, are not made available to the medical units, the admission procedure will have to be repeated, at least in part, by the individual medical units.

The acquired data are mainly used for patient identification (Section 5.1.3.7.1). Among these data are master data (name(s), birth date, address, sex), referring physician, insurance, and ward/ambulatory unit.

Definitions of the **master data** file vary. It sometimes includes only "personal data" and sometimes all data captured during admission.

The patient admission triggers several procedures, which are principally administrative, such as opening a patient account, initiating a medical record, assigning a hospital registration number, retrieving the medical record from the archive, or printing standard forms.

During a modern patient admission procedure data are input into a computer, resulting in two important consequences:

- Patient identification data are immediately available for other subsystems of the hospital information system (Section 6.3.2).
- During admission, access to historic patient data is possible (abbreviation of the admission procedure by adoption of already stored valid data; message to the archive for supply of the medical record; activation of important medical data such as "risks").

Most systems involve additional components such as

- patient appointment and summoning,
- transfer and discharge.

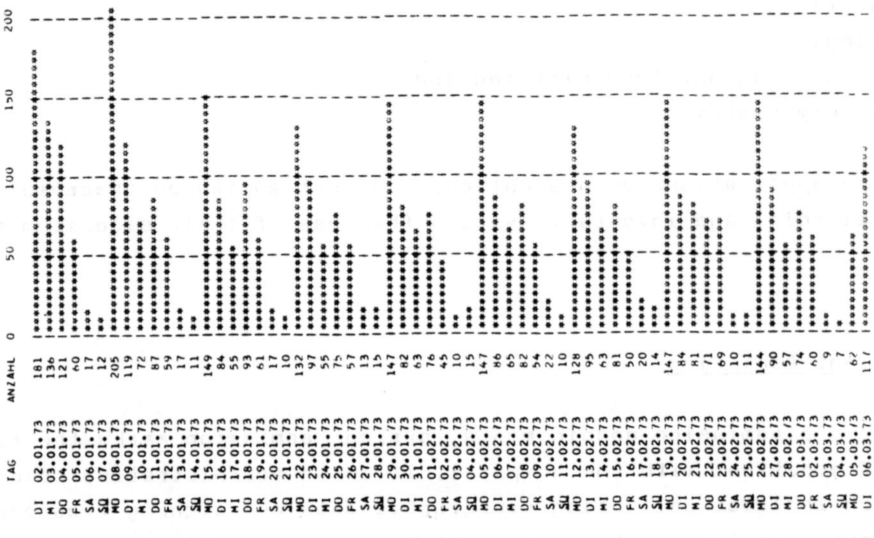

Fig. 6.4: Frequencies of patient admission in the Medical School Münster [85] (ANZAHL= frequency, TAG= calendar date)

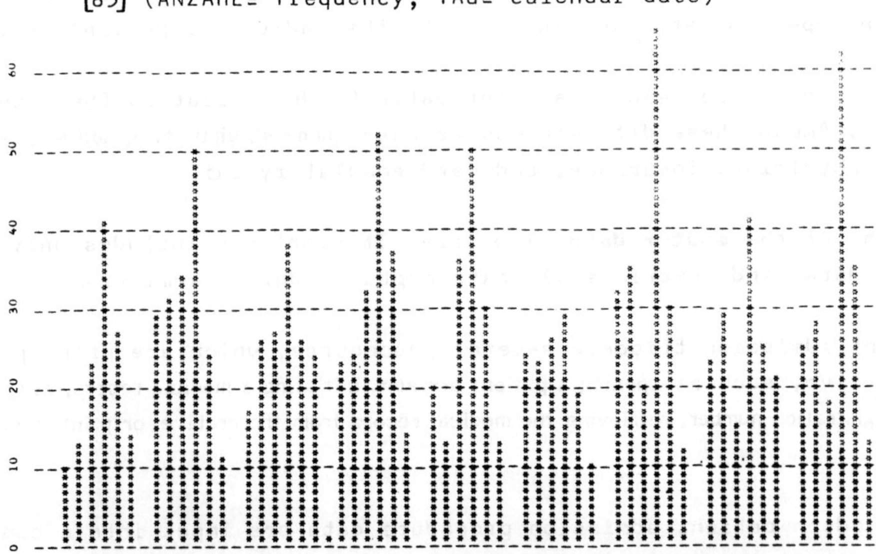

Fig. 6.5: Frequencies of request in the cytological laboratory of the Medical School Hannover [184] (ANZAHL=frequency, TAG=calendar date)

Surveys of the **occupancies** in a hospital are possible on the basis of the transfer and discharge data (admission journal, bed occupancy statistics, census).

Various systems and programs for patient admission are published. Most computer vendors offer "packages", which handle not only patient admission, but also patient accounting and billing.

The deviation from a Uniform Distribution of admissions over time (Fig. 6.4) complicates planning, because it results in a deviation from a Uniform Distribution of the workload in medical units (Fig. 6.5). This situation leads itself to an increased length of patient stay or a poor economical utilization of resources.

6.2.2 Inventory Systems

Variable amounts of a product may be stored (Fig. 6.6). The **stock** is used to meet the requirements (**demand**) of clients. It is **supplied** by purchase from a supplier. The **stockkeeping policy** both generates **costs** (costs for supply, stockkeeping, transport to clients, ...) and makes a **profit** by sale to a client.

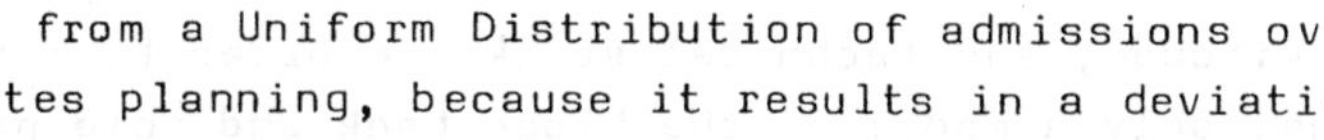

Fig. 6.6: Simple inventory system

Consider a **planning period** that is divided into **intervals**. The stockkeeping policy E determines the amount of supply to be purchased at the beginning of each interval. Therefore, the model distinguishes two types of variables:

- **state variables** describing the actual content of the stock, and
- **decision variables**, the determination of which represents the decision E.

For example, the "stock before supply" is a state variable and the "supply" is a decision variable. For determination of an optimal policy a target function Z(E) is used, which may be defined as the difference between gross income G(E) and costs C(E) (i.e., **net profit**):

$$Z(E) = G(E) - C(E) .$$

The optimal decision is that one, which maximizes net profits. Other optimization criteria are cost minimization and sales maximization.

The individual elements of the model are: stock structure, product structure, planning period, demand, supply, stock, decision space, and target function.

Medical stockkeeping problems are experienced particularly in the blood bank, pharmacy, kitchen, and technical stock. In order to introduce the essential notions, only a model of the blood bank and some peculiarities of the pharmacy are presented. Other stockkeeping problems are solved according to essentially the same principles.

6.2.2.1 Blood Bank

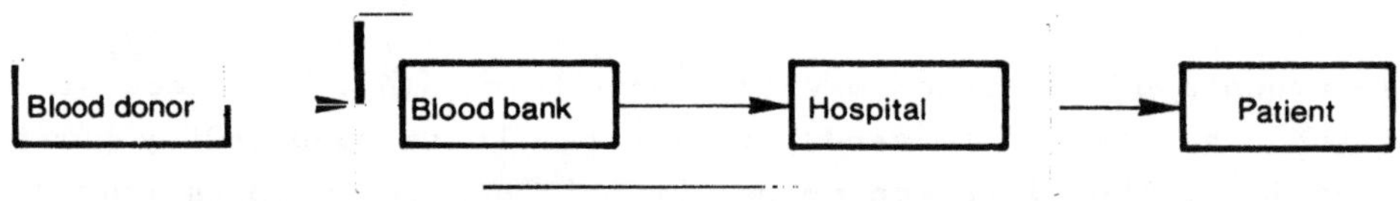

Fig. 6.7: Inventory system of a blood bank. The model is a 2-stage model if there is an intermediate stock in the hospital

The **stock structure** of a blood bank may be described by a 1-stage or a 2-stage model (Fig. 6.7).

The **product structure** comprises eight products, corresponding to the combinations of the four blood groups (A, B, AB, O) with the two levels of the rhesus factor (Rh+, Rh-). A patient needs a certain amount of one of these products. But the final decision about whether an ordered product can be used is made after delivery (tolerance test).

The products are perishable and cannot be kept in stock for an arbitrary long period. After exceeding the expiration date they can no longer be used for their usual purpose, but can be processed by pharmaceutic industry.

Planning period and **planning intervals** depend on the special inventory system. Intervals are in the magnitude of days or weeks.

The **demand** is determined by the attending physician. He orders the blood either directly from the blood bank (1-stage model) or from the hospital laboratory (2-stage model). Demand is partially known over a short period (e.g., planning of an operation), and partially unforeseeable (emergency). Demand is described by a probability function.

Demand always has to be supplied. If an item is out of stock, then the blood has to be ordered from a supplier (emergency blood donor, other stock), in principle without delay, and usually at higher costs.

Supply is normally obtained by voluntary blood donors either at regular intervals or spontaneously. Therefore, delivery to stock is also stochastic in contrast to most industrial inventory systems, because not every blood donor is always available or capable of making an acceptable donation.

Supply is the primary **decision variable**. Further decision variables are supply times and distribution in peripheral stocks (2-stage model). They determine the **stock**.

The **target function** primarily contains the **costs** for supply of blood ("regular" or emergency), stockkeeping, and transportation.

The **profit** results from selling the blood to a patient or to industry if out-dated. In the latter case the profit is smaller.

We now present an algorithm for the solution of a simplified problem. The planning period shall be divided into intervals with the limits t_i $(i=0,1,\dots,n)$. It is assumed that only one product has to be stored.

Stock shall be equal to α at the beginning of the k-th **interval** $(t_{k-1},t_k]$. The **demand** B_k shall be a random variable described by the probability function $f_k(b)$. α is not a random variable, because stock is known at time t_{k-1}.

The costs for **supply** of x_k units shall be the sum of fixed costs a_k and variable costs c_k depending on the amount of supply:

$$\delta_k\cdot\left(a_k + c_k(x_k)\right), \qquad \delta_k = \begin{cases} 1, & x_k > 0 \\ 0, & x_k \leq 0 \end{cases} .$$

Shortages have to be supplied with costs

$$d_k(\alpha+x_k-B_k).$$

For $\alpha+x_k-B_k \geq 0$ we have $d_k(\alpha+x_k-B_k)=0$. Considering the make-up of shortages, stock at beginning of the (k+1)-st interval is equal to

$$A_{k+1} = \max(0,\alpha+x_k-B_k).$$

Costs of **stockkeeping** depend only on stock:

$$g_k(\alpha+x_k).$$

The expected minimal costs for the intervals k to n are the sum of the minimal costs for interval k and the costs for intervals (k+1) to n. If an optimal decision is made, i.e., if the expected costs are minimized, then the minimal costs $Y_k(\alpha)$ for intervals k to n are:

$$Y_k(\alpha) = \min_{x_k}\left[\delta_k\cdot\big(a_k+c_k(x_k)\big)+ E\big(d_k(\alpha+x_k-B_k)\big)+ g_k(\alpha+x_k) + E\big(Y_{k+1}(A_{k+1})\big)\right].$$

In this formula, $E\big(Y_{k+1}(A_{k+1})\big)$ is the expectation of the costs for the intervals (k+1) to n when an optimal decision at the beginning of the (k+1)-st interval is made. It depends only on A_{k+1}. Therefore, one can start from the n-th interval and recursively compute the minimal costs for the k-th interval depending on the stock at the beginning of this interval. This class of problems belongs to the stochastic decision problems (Section 3.5).

If all aspects of the "blood bank" are considered, then the optimization problem becomes so complex that solutions have to be found by simulation. For example, we have to assume that the demands in the individual intervals are interrelated. The unknown probability distributions for demand, supply, and emergency have to be estimated by the corresponding frequency distributions.

If in a 2-stage model there is only a supply of the intermediate stocks by the central stock, then the model can be simplified to two 1-stage stocks.

However, this model is not optimal. If transportation costs have an essential influence on the costs, then supply of an intermediate stock should comprise blood of all blood groups, the stock of which approaches a predetermined lower bound. Furthermore, the probability of out-dating is decreased by moving "older" blood from a stock with low sales to a stock with higher sales.

These considerations illustrate that an inventory system for a blood bank must consider far more than a common industrial model:

- products are identified not only by their amounts, but have to be recorded individually (location, expiration date),
- the "suppliers" have to be recorded with additional data permitting statements concerning their availability (e.g., date of last blood donation),
- a transportation model in a 2-stage model has to ensure an economical exchangeability of blood among intermediate stocks.

Simulation results for three different models of a regional blood bank serving several hospitals with intermediate stocks (2-stage model) are contained in [116]. Costs could be reduced to one third.

6.2.2.2 Pharmacy

The pure stockkeeping problems of the pharmacy resemble industrial applications more than those of a blood bank. But more complex systems emerge when stockkeeping is related to medical problems (Section 6.3.2.2).

Pharmacy stocks in German hospitals usually have two stages, because the pharmacies keep intermediate stocks on wards, ambulatory units, and diagnostic units. In the United States the 1-stage model is becoming more common, where the patients are directly supplied from the pharmacy.

Inventory systems for the pharmacy are highly desirable for several reasons:

- the number of different drugs is very high,
- drugs differ only in the ratios of substances, but not in substances themselves,
- drugs differ only in name and price,
- drugs must be sold only before the specified expiration date,
- the ratio of drug costs to the total costs of health care is high,
- there are legal requirements that careful records be kept concerning the administration of certain (i.e., controlled) drugs (opiates, radionuclides).

6.3 Information Systems

Information systems contain individual **objects** related by defined relations, the **actions** of which are acquisition, storage, extraction, and representation of **information** (Chapter 5). Information systems are related to an **environment**, i.e., they themselves are objects (**subsystems**) of a larger system connected to the other objects by **interfaces** [98].

Thus, a laboratory information system is a subsystem of a hospital information system.

The relations to the environment have to be defined in order to ensure a smooth communication. The user is only interested in the **interface** problems addressed by this requirement, whereas the internal **architecture** of a computer-supported information system is of minor importance to him.

The following example demonstrates how strong decision support functions influence the design of an information system.

Suppose there is a simplified version of a computer-supported system for surveillance of **bed occupancy**, covering the bed plan of the hospital as well as each admission and discharge of a patient. If properly developed, the system will always be able to present valid data concerning the number of free beds.

However, in practice, the queries of a user become much more complex very quickly. For example, in addition to the report "10 beds free" it might be interesting to know why there are only 10 free beds. This question relates to the question of who occupies a certain bed and when a certain bed will presumably be free. Answering the last question may be quite complex and belongs to the area of decision support (is the state of a patient such that his discharge might be assumed after two days? If not, why not?).

This example illustrates a central problem of computer-supported information systems. The systems practically relevant for medicine are **dynamic** systems, which change their state depending on time. This dynamic aspect is also incorporated into the interfaces and the objects of the environment (information transmission to the outside world depends, for example, on the availability of the receiver).

Two additional influences have to be distinguished from these temporal changes:

- **Information requirements** of the outside world changes in reaction to a computer-supported information system. Even a most careful systems analysis cannot prevent some information, initially classified as essential, from never needed, or new specifications or requirements emerging soon after putting a system into operation.
- **Natural development** of the outside world results in new information and in new information requirements, for example, by developing new tests with new and so far unknown diagnostic possibilities.

6.3.1 Communication Systems

Basic to an information system is the transmission of messages. Therefore, information systems rest on a **communication system** comprising individual **stations** and connecting **communication lines** [78]. A station may be a **transmitter**, a **receiver**, and/or an **exchanger** of messages (Section 2.2.1).

A communication line can be **dedicated**, i.e., strictly assigned to a transmitter and a receiver, and it can be used in a single direction or in both directions. In addition, there are **general** communication lines used by more than one transmitter and/or receiver.

The **architecture** of a communication system rests on its functions for message transmission; in addition, it depends particularly on its **sensivity** to the failure of individual components, on its **extendability** by new components, and on its **costs** (Fig. 6.8):

- Each station in a **ring** is connected to two neighbors. The ring is relatively simple and easy to extend, but it is sensitive to the interruption of a connection. This is particularly true, when messages are only transmitted in a single direction.
- This disadvantage is not present in the **complete ring**, which, however, has high costs for extensions. Extension by an additional station requires establishing all connections to each one of the stations already present.
- The **bus** is a general communication line, whereby the source must obtain "control" of the line prior to message transmission. If the bus is interrupted, then all connections are interrupted.
- The **star** has a central exchanger. It is relatively simple and easily extendable. If the exchanger fails, then all connections fail.
- In the regular **net** each station is also exchanger and decides to whom an incoming message is to be transmitted. In general, the regular net combines the characteristics both of the complete ring and the star.

Complex communication systems may be hierarchically structured (Fig. 6.9). A frequently used principle is the local **concentrator**, which takes over the communication with other subsystems.

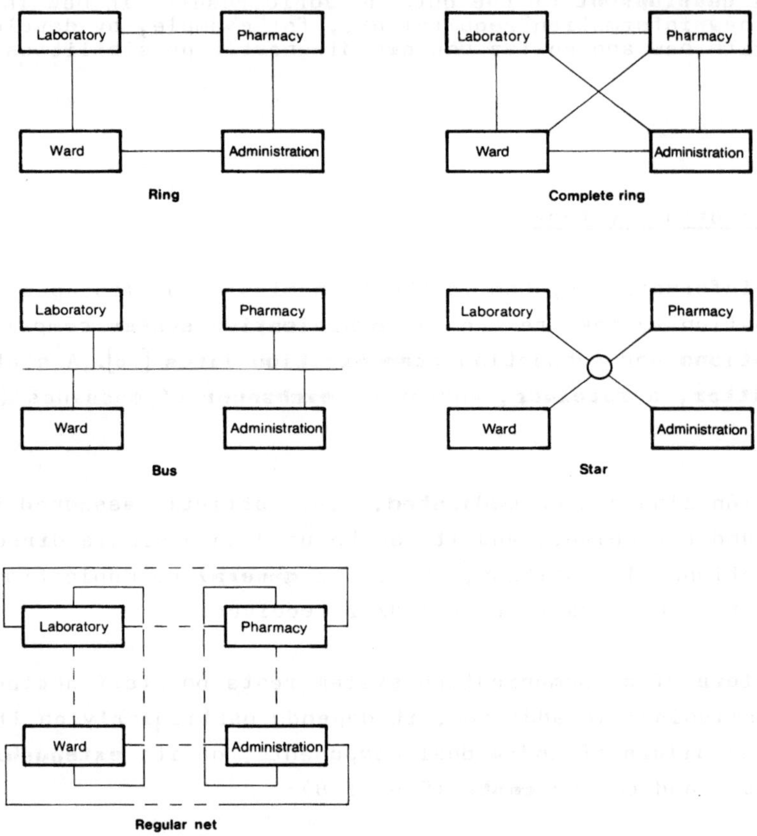

Fig. 6.8: Five models of a communication system with four stations

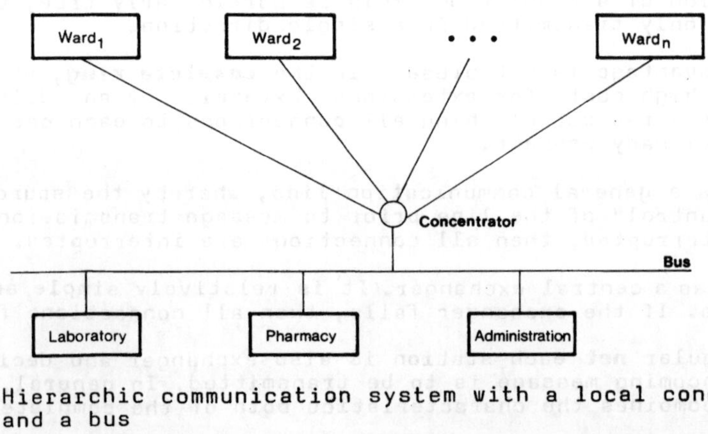

Fig. 6.9: Hierarchic communication system with a local concentrator and a bus

6.3.2 Hospital Information Systems (HIS)

At present, the definition of information systems is so general that the individual functions of an HIS are not specified. Therefore, very different systems are described in the literature, which are called HIS.

A first structure is derived from the structure of a hospital:

Patient care	**Functional unit**	**Supply**	**Administration**
wards ambulatory units	laboratories radiology nuclear medicine ECG-unit ---	pharmacy blood bank technical stock kitchen ---	admission accounting billing ---

These four areas are completed by **research** and **teaching** in university hospitals.

6.3.2.1 Objectives of a Hospital Information System

Patient data are the source of all activities in a hospital. Because data captured at a certain station are needed by other stations in order to do their tasks, data acquisition, input, storage, retrieval, and transmission must be organized.

The most important objectives of an HIS are:

- improvement of information,
- acceleration of presentation of information,
- rationalization of course of operations,
- relief from routine work,
- decision support.

Frequently, these objectives result in competing requirements. Thus, optimization of diagnostic and therapeutic procedures for an individual patient, on the one hand, and optimization of hospital organization, on the other hand, do not necessarily have the same consequences.

Essentially, an HIS should satisfy the requirements resulting from the increasing differentiation and the increasing amount of data. But we must not forget that computer support of a communication system concerns only message transmission. Therefore, improvement of information systems has additional aspects, the disregard of which cannot be balanced by technical means.

The communication systems of the hospitals, as developed in the past, are ineffective and unreliable. A real improvement of quality, and not merely treatment of superficial symptoms, will only be attained by a fundamental reorganization of information flow.

Surprisingly, perhaps, **cost reduction** has not been mentioned as an important objective of an HIS. This objective is frequently listed in the literature, particularly when addressed to political financing. But a computer-supported HIS is so multi-faceted and has such deep influences on patient care and hospital structure that, at present, "cost reduction" is only a catchword.

Development and employment of an HIS should contribute principally to medicine in meeting the increasing requirements. Introduction of new technologies, which may be compared with this area, has almost never resulted in primary cost reduction. At the time automated telephone exchange was introduced, manual exchange was cheaper. But automated exchange presented the prerequisite for the enormous growth of the telephone net, which would otherwise have been impossible or significantly more costly.

If the above-mentioned objectives are taken seriously, then it is often no question whether computer support is cheaper than manual operations, but whether one is willing to pay for it, because there is frequently no manual alternative. After all, the cheapest hospital is still a hospital without patients. Economical operation (whatever that is) is desirable, but decisions concerning an HIS must not merely be made on the basis of costs, which are frequently not even measurable.

There are many possibilities for **rationalization** of the operations in a hospital. But there are also instances for non-technologic marginal conditions obstructing rationalization.

A frequently mentioned objective of an HIS is shortening of patient stay in the hospital. This may be very sensible for the individual patient and for the national economy. However, it may not be very economical for an individual hospital, when the hospital is paid for days and not for services, because a short hospital stay generates higher daily costs than a longer stay.

Improvement of information can be obtained in several ways. Reducing the frequency of data acquisition - in the optimal case each datum is acquired only once - reduces the frequency of errors. Information extraction by aggregating data from different sources improves the potential for analysis.

A typical example is the presentation of important information from patient history, already triggered by admission ("risks" such as allergies or continuous therapies).

The **complete ring** or the **net** (Section 6.3.1) approach the traditional hospital structure best. They are favored by the direct connection of individual stations, because the risk of communication disturbances increases with the number of exchangers. A further advantage is the fact that discounting a communication line concerns only the stations directly involved, whereas all other lines may still work. These are important considerations to be kept in mind when the fascinating advantages of a star are considered.

In a **star** the data are nearly all centralized and can be integrated in an optimal way. Multiple storage of data can be eliminated, whereas in a complete ring data must be stored in each node, because each station must have access to a subset of the master data in order to relate the data to the patient. This results in serious problems especially concerning data update.

For example, if after termination of the admission procedure it appears that the name has to be corrected, then in a complete ring the correcting station must ensure that each false copy is corrected in each station storing this datum.

This problem has not yet been solved with justifiable expenses and sufficient safety for large systems such as are needed in hospitals.

In contrast to this, a single correction in the central data base suffices in a star in order to present the correct datum to each station.

The optimal architecture will be hierarchic. Each station must make available certain "local" data, which are also of interest to other stations. Therefore, the compromise between local independence with regard to data acquisition, update, and retrieval, on the one hand, and dependence on other stations or on a central data base, on the other hand, determines the architecture of a system in practice.

6.3.2.2 Functions of a Hospital Information System

At present, there is no HIS meeting the above-described objectives sufficiently well. But subsystems have been developed and have demonstrated potential fundamental solutions of the problems. The most important functions are:

- patient admission, bed occupancy, appointment scheduling,
- acquisition of service requests and presentation of planning foundations for the service units,
- service acquisition, accounting, and billing,
- inventory systems,
- menu-planning,
- result acquisition and evaluation (clinical laboratory, nuclear medicine, ECG, ...),
- automated medical reporting,
- documentation and archive administration,
- decision support,
- administrative functions (accounting, property management, financial accounts, ...).

They are presented in detail in the voluminous special literature and in the preceding sections.

This list omits functions referred to as research and teaching. These should be conceptually separated from an HIS, even if they utilize data of the hospital organization (e.g., teaching programs utilizing "actual" data). If all computer applications in a hospital are interpreted as components of an HIS, then finally the publication of national statistics belongs to an HIS. But then the concept becomes so vague that it no longer means anything.

The multiple relations and the several possible realizations are explained by means of an example (Fig. 6.10).

Drug therapy as a component of a computer-supported HIS can be interpreted as pure a **documentation** problem, where for each patient all therapies are stored for later statistical evaluation.

When therapy is relevant for **accounting**, there is an additional relation to administration, to which the therapy (including price) has to be transmitted.

Because knowledge of the therapy may be relevant for the evaluation of findings, this information is additionally made available to selected service units. Thus, evaluation of an ECG (cardiac drugs) or of laboratory results, detection of micro-organisms and their sensitivities in microbiology (antibiotics), and planning of operations (anticoagulants) depend on the knowledge of the therapy.

A reliable organization of drug administration on the **wards** is supported by work lists (patient, time, drug, dosage).

The system could be required to **check** the plausibility of prescriptions (invalid dosage), to offer cheaper alternatives for expensive drugs, and to indicate possible interactions (inhibition, cumulation, incompatibility) to the attending physician.

There are additional relations to a **drug stock** on the wards, to an inventory system in the pharmacy, etc.

For certain therapies the patient has to be educated. Therefore, there are relations to **teaching programs** for patients.

Thus, the functions related to the data concerning drug therapy may become arbitrarily voluminous and complex.The example illustrates how precisely these functions have to be specified before a computer-supported HIS is developed.

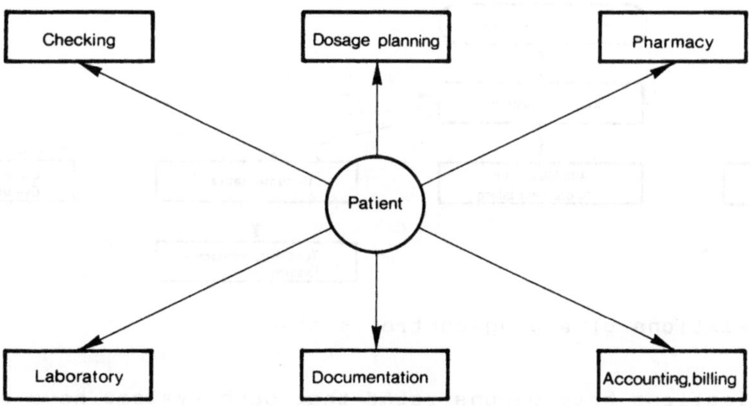

Fig. 6.10: Relations among data concerning drug therapy

The central component of an HIS is the **data base** (Section 5.1.1). It is updated by data input via interfaces (Section 5.2). The structure depends on type and number of observed attributes and, in particular, on the permitted access paths. But these paths usually differ in data input and retrieval. While data input is almost always patient-oriented, retrieval has different structuring criteria such as time, location, specialty, source, method of data capture, or attribute values.

Therefore, an HIS has intimate relations to documentation systems. The mixture of objectives of an HIS and a documentation system is the most frequent cause of misplanning and failure.

6.3.2.3 Drug-Control Systems

A drug-control system (Fig. 6.11) is an important subsystem of an HIS. Acquisition of **drug prescriptions** can support decision making under different aspects, like checking of indication, dosage, and application form, or warning of drug interactions.

Worksheets may be printed to support patient care including patient, time, and medication.

Acquisition of **drug administration** affects nearly all areas of a hospital (Section 6.3.2.2).

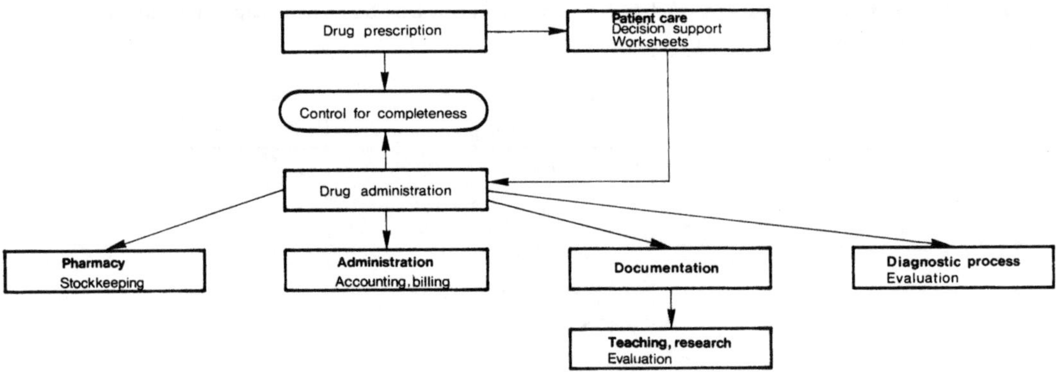

Fig. 6.11: Relations of a drug-control system

Several applications have demonstrated that such systems have cost-reducing side-effects, which can only be partially derived from the optimization of stockkeeping. A large part is the result of optimizing physician behavior. Many hospitals have already established a drug committee. A drug-control system practically enforces such a committee. The very first effect is the reduction of the drug spectrum kept in stock.

As it happens, many drugs are in stock only, because individual physicians believe that these drugs are especially effective or do not know an alternative. Sometimes, these physicians have already left the hospital but the dormant stock remained.

Indication lists containing only those drugs whose effects are known and which are the cheapest alternatives reduce the costs significantly. Nevertheless, **justifiable** deviations from the lists may be permitted.

6.3.2.4 Peculiarities in a Hospital Information System

The discussion of peculiarities in an HIS is frequently more emotional than realistic. One extreme is the "materialistic" viewpoint, which assumes that an HIS is not significantly different from a management information system as it can be implemented in a bank. The "humanistic" viewpoint constitutes the other extreme, postulating that data processing in medicine has peculiarities requiring not only special software but also special hardware. In recent years, financial considerations have swung the pendulum towards the materialistic extreme.

From the technologic viewpoint, patient admission is, in principle, merely opening an account. Differences emerge in exceptional cases. Thus, "opening an account" in a hospital must be possible without the "holder" of the account being fully identified (irresponsive patient) or without having a guarantee (emergency).

Data and relations are much more complex than in established management information systems. Most of the relations are not operationally defined. But a computer-supported HIS oughts to stimulate improvement in exactly this area and should contribute to the acceleration of its development.

Some further important non-technical aspects for the understanding of the problems are:

- The conventional system has emerged over a long period and has resulted in an organizational and personal structure, which is anything but reliable even under conventional conditions.
- There are psychologic and sociologic problems of medical and paramedical personnel, which can only be solved by education and "acclimatization".
- Personnel is frequently under a stress, sometimes being so strong, that disturbances are not tolerated, especially when caused by technical devices.
- There are many exceptional cases where for most components completeness of data cannot be a prerequisite for operation.
- Precise authorization with respect to organizational decisions is missing or unproperly distributed.
- Complexity of problems and lack of experience lead to long developmental periods and unreliable hardware and software.

- Half-hearted decisions require development without adequate resources in equipment and personnel (requirement for "transportable" solutions in an immature state; development of systems for routine use on computer systems, which are primarily available for research and teaching).

6.4 Disease Registers

Disease registers are important for epidemiology and patient care.

Epidemiology aims at the detection of the influences on the incidences of diseases. Therefore, the data base must contain not only personal data but also diagnoses in sufficiently detailed differentiation as well as the values of potential influences (attributes). Because for these investigations the set of potential influences is open, such systems are generally not suited for the detection of causes but "only" for hypothesis generation. Subsequently, these hypotheses have to be tested in controlled clinical trials.

In **patient care** disease registers are important for chronic diseases, especially if diagnostic processes and therapy are distributed among several stations. Among these registers, **cancer registry** has become especially well-known [39,40,158]. These registers enforce a documentation with the greater reliability and completeness, which is intended to compensate for the insufficiencies of the medical record (Section 5.1.3.1).

In practice, disease registers are frequently required for epidemiologic investigations as well as for patient care. This can easily result in conflicting objectives. The amount of data to be acquired is soon so large that completeness is no longer assured.

The most important objectives are:

- detecting local and patient-related influences on incidences,
- clarifying the relation between disease course (in particular survival time), diagnosis, and therapy,
- comparing the effectiveness of different therapies,
- standardizing therapies,
- improving the health care system by detecting causes of delays in diagnostic and therapeutic processes,
- improving follow-up procedures.

The two main types of disease registers are **population-oriented** registers primarily for epidemiologic purposes and **hospital-oriented** registers primarily for patient care.

In the absence of information standards, different registers are usually incompatible. Therefore, the World Health Organization has published rules to ensure a minimal compatibility [190].

6.5 Bibliographies

Not only physicians working in research are interested in specialized bibliographies [36]. The rapid development of medicine has resulted in a far-reaching specialization and a plethora of publications, from which even an expert sees only a small excerpt in his special area.

Specialization is only one item among several causes of this phenomenon, which everybody complains about. An additional cause is a widely-accepted false criterion for judging scientific productivity. The process starts with habilitation, where the preceding scientific activity is measured by the **number** of papers and not by a rational judgement of **quality.** This behavior is often continued in later scientific activity and results in the bad habit of publishing the same results, acquired by a scientific team, in several papers with minor modifications, permuting the order of the authors.

These defects can at least in part be balanced by bibliographies. They maintain data bases containing abstracts of relevant papers. Besides the usual bibliographic data such as authors, periodical, year, and title, mainly an index of the content is stored (Section 5.4.1).

These operations, mostly manual, require large and highly trained human resources. Because of high costs, bibliographies are frequently financed by public corporations and are centrally employed.

The data base is either evaluated at regular intervals or is used to answer spontaneous queries concerning relevant literature. Advanced systems permit spontaneous queries in a dialog with the user.

The best-known bibliographies are provided by the National Library of Medicine (NLM) in Bethesda, Maryland. The thesaurus used is "Medical Subject Headings" (MeSH). It is also available online.

MEDLARS (MEDical Literature And Retrieval System) has become the starting point for several specialized bibliographies, most of which are not only regularly published (see INDEX MEDICUS), but are also available online. Some bibliographies are also available in Europe [96]. The most important specializations are:

- MEDLINE (biomedical literature from 3,000 periodicals and selected monographs),
- TOXLINE (toxicology, pharmacology),
- CANCERLINE (malignant tumors).

Bibliographies of the NLM are partially available in other countries. In Germany the "Deutsches Institut für Medizinische Dokumentation und Information" (DIMDI) in Cologne is responsible.

Another example is CANCERNET [188] with literature information concerning malignant tumors. In CANCERNET an international cooperation is realized.

7. References

1 AHO, A.V., ULLMAN, J.D.: The Theory of Parsing, Translation, and Compiling
Vol. I, II, London 1972/1973

2 AMERICAN NATIONAL STANDARDS INSTITUTE: American National Standard COBOL
X3. 23, 1974

3 AMERICAN NATIONAL STANDARDS INSTITUTE: FORTRAN
(ANSI X3. 9-1966 und X3. 10-1966)

4 ANDERSON, J.: Aims of Medical Information
In: [8], 22-27

5 ANDERSON, J.: Definition of Terms Used in Medical Information
In: [8], 14-21

6 ANDERSON, J. (Edt.): Medical Informatics Europe
Berlin, Heidelberg, New York 1978

7 ANDERSON, J., FORSYTHE, J.M.: MEDINFO 74
Amsterdam, Oxford, New York 1975

8 ANDERSON, J., FORSYTHE, J.M. (Edts): Information Processing of Medical Records
Amsterdam, Oxford, New York 1970

9 ANDERSON, T.W.: An Introduction to Multivariate Statistical Analysis
New York 1958

10 ARBEITSAUSSCHUSS MEDIZIN IN DER DGD: Ein dokumentationsgerechter Krankenblatt-
kopf für stationäre Patienten aller klinischen Fächer (sog. allgemeiner Krankenblattkopf)
Med. Dok. 5 (1961), 57-70

11 ASTRAHAN, M.M., CHAMBERLIN, D.D.: Implementation of a Structured English Query
Language
CACM 18 (1975), 580-588

12 BAILEY, N.T.J., THOMPSON, M. (Edts.): Systems Aspects of Health Planning
Amsterdam, Oxford, New York 1975

13 BAUER, F.L., EICKEL. J. (Edts.): Compiler Construction
Berlin, Heidelberg, New York 1976

14 BAUER, F.L., GOOS, G.: Informatik I
Berlin, Heidelberg, New York 1973

15 BIRKHOFF, G.: Lattice Theory
Providence, Rhode Island 1967

16 BLEICH, H.L.: Computer-Based Consultation - Electrolyte and Acid-Base Disorders
Amer. J. Med. 53 (1972), 285-291

17 BLITTERSDORF, F.: Krankenblattabschluß
In: [86], 443-452

18 BOCK, H.E., EGGSTEIN, M.: Automationsprobleme in der Medizin
Dtsch. Med. Wschr. 93 (1968), 985-990

19 BOLC, L. (Edt.): Natural Language Communication With Computers
Berlin, Heidelberg, New York 1978

20 BOLINGER, R.E., PRICE, S., KYNER, J.L.: Experience With Automation as an Aid in the
Management of Diabetes
Diabetes 22 (1973), 480-484

21 BRAUN, S.: Möglichkeiten und Probleme der Textverarbeitung auf linguistischer Grundlage
In: [182], 59-69

22 BRODMAN, K., ERDMANN, A.J., WOLFF, H.G.: Cornell Medical Index Health Questionnaire Manual
Cornell University Medical College, New York 1949

23 BUNDESMINISTER FÜR JUGEND, FAMILIE UND GESUNDHEIT (Edt.): Internationale Klassifikation der Krankheiten (ICD) 1979
Bonn 1979

24 CENTRAL HEALTH SERVICES COUNCIL: The Standardisation of Hospital Medical Records
H.M. Stat. Off., London No. 32-529, 1965

25 CHAMBERLIN, D.D., BOYCE, R.F.: SEQUEL: A Structured English Query Language
Proc. ACM-SIGFIDET Workshop Ann Arbor, Michigan, 1974, 249-264

26 CHARNIAK, E.: Inference and Knowledge 1
In: [27], 1-21

27 CHARNIAK, E., WILKS, Y. (Edts.): Computational Semantics
Amsterdam, Oxford, New York 1976

28 CIOMS (Council for International Organizations of Medical Sciences): Medical Terminology and Lexicography
Basel 1966

29 CIOMS (Council for International Organizations of Medical Sciences): Vorläufige Internationale Nomenklatur
Heidelberg 1973 ff.

30 CODD, E.F.: A Data Sublanguage Founded on the Relational Calculus
In: CODD, E.F., DEAN, A.L. (Edts.): ACM-SIGFIDET Workshop on Data Description, Access and Control, San Diego 1971, 35-68

31 CODD, E.F.: A Relational Model of Data for Large Shared Data Banks
CACM 13 (1970), 377-387

32 COLLEGE OF AMERICAN PATHOLOGISTS: Systematized Nomenclature of Pathology
Chicago, Ill. 1969

33 COLLEGE OF AMERICAN PATHOLOGISTS: Systematized Nomenclature of Medicine
Chicago, Ill. 1976

34 COLLEN, M.F.: General Requirements for a Medical Information System (MIS)
Comp. Biomed. Res. 3 (1970), 393-406

35 COLLEN, M.F. et al.: Reliability of a Self-Administered Medical Questionnaire
Arch. Intern. Med. 123 (1969), 664-681

36 DAY, M.S.: Survey of Health Bibliographical Information Systems
In: [150], 297-299

37 DEUTSCHSPRACHIGER TNM-AUSSCHUSS: Tumor-Lokalisations-Schlüssel
Deutschsprachiger TNM-Ausschuß 1974

38 DIETHELM, L.: Röntgendiagnostik, Strahlentherapie, Nuklearmedizin
In: [86], 791-840

39 DRUCKSACHE 7/4711 DES DEUTSCHEN BUNDESTAGES vom 9.2.1976

40 DRUCKSACHE 7/5459 DES DEUTSCHEN BUNDESTAGES vom 22.6.1976

41 DUDECK, J.: Die klinische Bedeutung der automatischen Phonokardiogrammauswertung
In: [143], 83-91

42 EISENBERG, P. (Edt.): Semantik und künstliche Intelligenz
Berlin, New York 1977

43 ENDRES, A.: Analyse und Verifikation von Programmen
Munich, Vienna 1977

44 ENGELBRECHT, R.: MHBS: Das Mineralhaushalt-Bilanzierungssystem
In: HEITE, H.J. (Edt.): Krankenhausinformationssysteme. Erstrebtes und Erreichtes
Stuttgart, New York 1972

45 FELDMANN, U., REICHERTZ, P.L., SAUTER, K.: On the Selectivity of the Identification Number in the Patient Data Base of the Medical System Hannover
Meth. Inform. Med. 19 (1980), 28-26

46 FERMANIAN, J., MORICE, V.: Computerized Detection of Doubtful Data: A New Method
In: [150], 701-703

47 FISCHER, R.: Schreibfehlerkorrektur in Texten
Berlin, Heidelberg, New York 1980

48 FLEISCHER, W.: Wortbildung der deutschen Gegenwartssprache
Tübingen 1975

49 FORTRAN: Clarification of FORTRAN Standards - Initial Progress
CACM 12 (1969), 289-294

50 FORTRAN: Clarification of FORTRAN Standards - Second Report
CACM 14 (1971), 628-642

51 GERNET, H., OSTHOLT, H., WERNER, H.: Intraoculare Optik in Klinik und Praxis
Berlin 1978

52 GESELLSCHAFT FÜR KLASSIFIKATION e.V. (Edt.): Prinzipien der Klassifikation
Frankfurt 1977

53 GORDON, B.L.: Biomedical Language for Manual and Computer Applications
Meth. Inform. Med. 7 (1963), 5-7

54 GORDON, B.L. (Edt.): Current Medical Information and Terminology (CMIT)
Chicago, Ill. 1971

55 GORRY, G.A., BARNETT, G.O.: Experience With a Model of Sequential Diagnosis
Comput. Biomed. Res. 1 (1968), 490-507

56 GRAYBILL, F.A.: Theory and Application of the Linear Model
North Scitnate, Mass. 1976

57 GRIESSER, G. (Edt.): Realization of Data Protection in Health Information Systems
Amsterdam, Oxford, New York 1977

58 GROSS, R.: Medizinische Diagnostik - Grundlagen und Praxis
Berlin, Heidelberg, New York 1969

59 HADLEY, G.: Nichtlineare und dynamische Programmierung
Würzburg, Vienna 1969

60 HARTMANN, F.: Anamnese
In: Fischer-Lexikon Medizin 1, Frankfurt 1959

61 HARTMANN, F.: Die Anamnese (Teil I)
Klin. Gegenw. 10 (1965), 691-718

62 HARTMANN, F.: Elemente des ärztlichen Erkenntnisprozesses
In: [133], 390-418

63 HEAULME, M. de: Artificial Medical Languages, a Solution for Clinical Needs in Documentation. Example Using Remede System
In: [6], 63-71

64 HEINECKE, A. et al.: Praktische Übungen Biomathematik
Schriftenreihe des Instituts für Medizinische Informatik und Biomathematik der Univ. Münster, Heft 2, 1975

65 HERMES, H.: Einführung in die Mathematische Logik
Stuttgart 1976

66 HUANG, T.S. (Edt.): Picture Processing and Digital Filtering
Berlin, Heidelberg, New York 1975

67 HULTSCH, E.: Formale Beschreibung von Merkmalsstrukturen
Inaug. Diss., Münster 1981

68 IBM: PL/I Language Specifications
IBM Form-Number GY33-6003, 1970

69 IMMICH, H.: Klinischer Diagnosenschlüssel (KDS)
Stuttgart, New York 1966

70 IMMICH, H.: Praktische Anwendung der Klassifikations- und Codierungsprinzipien
In: [86], 245-266

71 IMMICH, H., WAGNER, G.: Basisdokumentation in der Klinik
In: [86], 335-376

72 INGELS, F.M.: Information and Coding Theory
Scranton 1971

73 JACOB, W., SCHEIDA, D., WINGERT, F.: Tumor-Histologie-Schlüssel
Berlin, Heidelberg, New York 1978

74 JANAS, J.M.: Automatic Recognition of Part-of-Speech for English Texts
Inf. Proc. Man. 13 (1977), 205-213

75 JELLIFFE, R.W., BUELL, J., KALABA, R.: Reduction of Digitalis Toxicity by Computer-Assisted Glycoside Dosage Regimens
Anns. Intern. Med. 77 (1972), 891-906

76 JUSTEN, M.R.: Die Dokumentation der Traumatologie am mittleren Krankenhaus
Inaug. Diss., Bochum 1970

77 KÜNKEL, H.: Quantitative EEG-Analyse und klinische Diagnostik. Stand und Perspektiven
In: [143], 92-103

78 KÄSTNER, H.: Architektur und Organisation digitaler Rechenanlagen
Stuttgart 1978

79 KILIAN, W., PORTH, A.J. (Edts.): Juristische Probleme der Datenverarbeitung in der Medizin
Berlin, Heidelberg, New York 1979

80 KNEDEL, M.: Datenverarbeitung im klinisch-chemischen Institut
Erlangen 1971

81 KNEDEL, M., KILLIAN, K.P.: Das automatisierte Laborsystem im Städt. Krankenhaus München-Harlaching - Funktion und Wirtschaftlichkeit
In: [143], 113-119

82 KNUTH, D.E.: The Art of Computer Programming, Vol. I
Reading, Mass. 1973

83 KOEPPE, P.: Zum Problem der EDV-gerechten Erfassung medizinischer Befunde
Meth. Inform. Med. 10 (1971), 25-29

84 KOEPPE, P. et al.: Das System ORVID. Ein Beitrag zur programmierten Dokumentation in der Röntgendiagnostik
Fortschr. Röntgenstr. Nukl. Med. 112 (1970), 103-110

85 KOLLEGIUM BIOMATHEMATIK NW: Biomathematik für Mediziner
Berlin, Heidelberg, New York 1976

86 KOLLER, S., WAGNER, G. (Edts.): Handbuch der medizinischen Dokumentation und Datenverarbeitung
Stuttgart, New York 1975

87 KOSSMANN, C.E. et al.: Recommendations for Standardization of Leads and of Specifications for Instruments in Electrocardiography and Vectorcardiography
Circulation 35 (1967), 583-602

88 KRAUTH, J., LIENERT, G.A.: KFA. Die Konfigurationsfrequenzanalyse
Freiburg, Munich 1973

89 KUHLENDAHL, H. et al.: Untersuchungen über die Schwerkrankenüberwachung mit DV-Anlagen
In: [143], 25-34

90 KURVER, P.H.J. et al.: Storage and Processing Obstetric Signals
In: [150], 1005-1009

91 LACHENBRUCH, P.A.: Discriminant Analysis
New York 1975

92 LAMSON, B.G.: Natural Language Retrieval System, Pathology Thesaurus
Los Angeles 1970

93 LEHMANN, E.L.: Testing Statistical Hypotheses
New York 1970

94 LEIBER, B.: Dokumentation der klinischen Syndrome
In: [86], 1349-1372

95 LEIBER, B., OLBRICH, G.: Die klinischen Syndrome
Munich, Berlin, Vienna 1972/73

96 LEITER, J.: On-Line Systems of the National Library of Medicine
In: [150], 349-353

97 LEWIS, S.M., BURGESS, B.J.: Quality Control in Haematology: Report of Interlaboratory Trials in Britain
Brit. Med. J. 4 (1969), 253-256

98 LOCKEMANN, P.C., MAYR, H.C.: Rechnergestützte Informationssysteme
Berlin, Heidelberg, New York 1978

99 LODWICK, G.S.: Better Interpretation and Reporting of Radiant Images
In: [150], 575-583

100 LODWICK, G.S. et al.: "ODARS", A Computer Aided System for Diagnosing and Reporting. Part I: Clinical Problems
In: HAENE, R. de, WAMBERSIE, A. (Edts.): Computers in Radiology
Basel 1970, 279-282

101 MÖHR, J.R.: Computer Assisted Medical History
Habilitation Thesis, Medizinische Hochschule Hannover 1976

102 MARTIN, J.M. et al.: Automatic Printing in Clear Language of Complete Medical Observations
In: [150], 293-295

103 MAULBETSCH, R.H.: Das Diagnostik-Informationssystem (DIS) der Medizinischen Universitätsklinik Tübingen
In: [168], 17-25

104 McCARTHY, J. et al.: LISP 1.5 Programmer's Manual
Cambridge, Mass. 1962

105 MICHAELIS, J.: Verschlüsselungssysteme in der Elektrokardiographie
In: [86], 719-726

106 MURNAGHAN, J.H., WHITE, K.L. (Edts.): Hospital Discharge Data
Report of the Conference on Hospital Discharge Abstract Systems
Med. Care 8, No. 4 (Suppl.) 1970

107 NACKE, O., GERDEL, W.: Terminologie, Klassifikation und Verschlüsselung
In: [86], 213-232

108 NIEMANN, H.: Mustererkennung - Einführung und Übersicht
Informatik-Spektrum 2 (1979), 12-24

109 NILSSON, N.J.: Artificial Intelligence
In: ROSENFELD, J.L. (Edt.): Information Processing 74
Amsterdam, Oxford, New York 1974, 778-801

110 NOMINA ANATOMICA
Amsterdam 1977

111 OSADA, N.: Beiträge zur Strukturanalyse der medizinischen Sprache
Inaug. Diss., Münster 1981

112 PÖPPL, S.J. et al.: Adaptive Nonlinear Approaches to Nonparametric Classification and Discrimination Techniques Based on Pipberger ECG-File
In: [150], 1017-1021

113 PACAK, M.G., DUNHAM, G.S.: Computers and Medical Language
Med. Inform. 4 (1979), 13-27

114 PACAK, M.G., NORTON, L.M., DUNHAM, G.S.: Morphosemantic Analysis of -ITIS Forms in Medical Language
Meth. Inform. Med. 19 (1978), 99-105

115 PACAK, M.G., PRATT, A.W.: Identification and Transformation of Terminal Morphemes in Medical English. Part II
Meth. Inform. Med. 17 (1978), 95-100

116 PAGE, B.: Testing Alternative Inventory Policies for a Regional Blood Bank
In: [6], 403-412

117 PASCHER, W., ROST, K., SCHEIBE, O.: Basisdokumentation in der Poliklinik
In: [86], 377-390

118 PERCY, C.L., BERG, J.W., THOMAS, L.B (Edts.): Manual of Tumor Nomenclature and Coding
American Cancer Society 1968

119 PIPBERGER, H.V.: Elektrokardiographie, Elektroenzephalographie und andere Registriermethoden
In: [86], 703-718

120 PIPBERGER, H.V. et al.: Recommendations for Standardization of Instruments in Electrocardiography and Vectorcardiography
IEEE Trans. Biomed. Engin. BME-14 (1967), 60-68

121 PORTH, A.J.: Laboratoriumsdaten
In: [86], 662-701

122 PORTH, A.J.: Untersuchungen und Verfahren zur Plausibilitätskontrolle im computer-unterstützten klinisch-chemischen Laboratorium
Habilitation Thesis, Medizinische Hochschule Hannover 1976

123 PRATT, A.W.: Medicine, Computers and Linguistics
Adv. Biomed. Engin. 3 (1973), 97-140

124 PRATT, A.W., PACAK, M.: Identification and Transformation of Terminal Morphemes in Medical English
Meth. Inform. Med. 8 (1969), 84-90

125 PRESTON, K., ONOE, M. (Edts.): Digital Processing of Biomedical Images
New York, London 1976

126 PREWITT, J.M.S.: New Vistas in Medical Reconstruction Imagery
In: [125], 133-160

127 PREWITT, J.M.S.: Object Enhancement and Extraction
In: LIPKIN, B.S., ROSENFELD, A. (Edts.): Picture Processing and Psychopictorics
New York 1970, 75-149

128 PROPPE, A., WAGNER, G.: Über die Zuverlässigkeit medizinischer Dokumente und Befunde
Med. Sachverständ. 52 (1956), 122-127

129 RÖTTGER, P. et al.: Konzeption und Organisation des AGK-Thesaurus
In: SIEMENS AG (Edt.): Symposium über Klartextanalyse in der Medizin (1)
Erlangen 1975, 52-60

130 RAWLINSON, F.: Semantische Untersuchung zur medizinischen Krankheitsterminologie
Marburg 1974

131 REALLEXIKON DER MEDIZIN
Munich, Berlin, Vienna 1977

132 REICHERTZ, P.L.: Informationssysteme in der Medizin
Bad Godesberg 1975

133 REICHERTZ, P.L., GOOS, G. (Edts.): Informatics and Medicine
Berlin, Heidelberg, New York 1977

134 ROSENFELD, A.: Picture Processing by Computer
Technical Report 68-71, Univ. of Maryland 1968

135 ROSENFELD,A., PARK, C.M., STRONG, J.P.: Noise Cleaning in Binary-Valued Digital Pictures Using "Propagation" Processes
Technical Report 69-91, Univ. of Maryland 1969

136 ROSENFELD, A., THOMAS, R.B., LEE, Y.H.: Edge and Curve Enhancement in Digital Pictures
Technical Report 69-93, Univ. of Maryland 1969

137 SAGER, N.: Natural Language Information Processing
New York 1981

138 SAGER, W.: Ein Programmsystem zur Prüfung von Klartextdaten in der dezentralen Datenerfassung
In: [182], 153-159

139 SALOMAA, A.K.: Formale Sprachen
Berlin, Heidelberg, New York 1978

140 SCHEFFÉ, H.: The Analysis of Variance
New York 1970

141 SCHEIBE, O.-A., WAGNER, G.: Die TNM-Klassifikation der malignen Tumoren
Wissenschaft und Praxis 23 (1975), 1767-1770

142 SCHLAGETER, G., STUCKY, W.: Datenbanksysteme: Konzepte und Modelle
Stuttgart 1977

143 SCHNEIDER, B., SCHÖNENBERGER, R. (Edts.): Datenverarbeitung im Gesundheitswesen
Berlin, Heidelberg, New York 1976

144 SCHNEIDER, W., SAGVALL HEIN, A.-L. (Edts.): Computational Linguistics in Medicine
Amsterdam, Oxford, New York 1977

145 SCHOTT, G.: Automatische Deflexion unter Verwendung eines Minimal-Wörterbuchs
Institut für Informatik der TU München, Nr. 7514, 1975

146 SCHWILL, W.D., WEIBEZAHN, R.: Einführung in die Programmiersprache BASIC
Braunschweig 1976

147 SCOTTISH HOME AND HEALTH DEPARTMENT: Hospital Medical Records in Scotland. Development and Standardisation
H.M. Stat. Off., Edinburgh No. 49-587, 1967

148 SCRAGG, G.: Semantic Nets as Memory Models
In: [27], 101-127

149 SHANNON, C.E., WEAVER, W.: The Mathematical Theory of Communication
Univ. of Illinois Press 1949

150 SHIRES, D.B., WOLF, H. (Edts.): MEDINFO 77
Amsterdam, Oxford, New York 1977

151 SHORTLIFFE, E.H.: Computer-Based Medical Consultations: MYCIN
New York 1976

152 SLACK, W.V., VAN CURA, L.J.: Patient Reaction to Computer-Based Medical Interviewing
Comp. Biomed. Res. 1 (1968), 527-531

153 SLAGLE, J.R., LEE, C.T.: Application of Game Tree Searching Techniques to Sequential Pattern Recognition
CACM 14 (1971), 103-110

154 SNEATH, P.H.A., SOKAL, R.R.: Numerical Taxonomy
San Francisco 1963

155 STANGE, K.: BAYES-Verfahren
Berlin, Heidelberg, New York 1977

156 STEINHAUSEN, D., LANGER, K.: Clusteranalyse
Berlin, New York 1977

157 SWOBODA, A. et al.: Rechnerunterstützte postoperative Intensivmedizin der Herz- und Gefäßchirurgie
In: [143], 35-41

158 SZUWART, U.: Vorbereitung zum Aufbau eines Krebsregisters
Schriftenreihe des Instituts für Medizinische Informatik und Biomathematik der Univ. Münster, Heft 3, 1977

159 TANENBAUM, A.S.: A Tutorial on ALGOL 68
ACM Computing Surveys 8 (1976), 155-190

160 THOMPSON, E.T., HAYDEN, A.D. (Edts.): Standard Nomenclature of Diseases and Operations
New York 1961

161 TURING, A.: Computing Machinery and Intelligence
Mind (1951), 1-17

162 U.S. NATIONAL COMMITTEE ON VITAL AND HEALTH STATISTICS: Uniform Hospital Abstract: Minimum Basic Data Set
U.S. Dept. H.E.W. Public Health Service Publication
Vital and Health Statistics Series 4 - No. 14, Rockville, Md. 1972

163 UICC (International Union Against Cancer): Illustrated Tumor Nomenclature
Berlin, Heidelberg, New York 1969

164 UICC (International Union Against Cancer): TNM Classification of Malignant Tumors
Geneva 1974

165 VAN WIJNGAARDEN, A. et al.: Revised Report on the Algorithmic Language ALGOL 68
Acta Informatica 5 (1975), 1-236

166 VOSSEPOEL, A.M.: Compliance Aspects of a Computer Assisted Anticoagulation Control System
In: [6], 651-656

167 WAGNER, G.: Datenkontrolle
In: [86], 267-288

168 WAGNER, G. (Edt.): Laboratory Information Systems. Hospital Pharmacy Systems
Stuttgart, New York 1978

169 WAGNER, G., NEWCOMBE, H.B.: Record Linkage. Its Methodology and Application in Medical Data Processing. A Bibliography
Meth. Inform. Med. 9 (1970), 121-138

170 WAGNER, G., STUTZER, G.: Über die Selektivität der sog. I-Zahl im "allgemeinen Krankenblattkopf" und die Brauchbarkeit ihrer einzelnen Komponenten
Meth. Inform. Med. 2 (1963), 148-155

171 WARNER, H.R.: Computer-Assisted Medical Decision-Making
London 1979

172 WARNER, H.R., TORONTO, A.F., VEASY, L.G.: Experience with BAYES' Theorem for Computer Diagnosis of Congenital Heart Disease
Anns. N.Y. Acad. Sci. 115 (1964), 558-567

173 WEDEKIND, H.: Datenbanksysteme I
Zurich 1974

174 WEDEKIND, H.: Systemanalyse
Munich 1973

175 WEED, L.L.: Medical Records, Medical Education and Patient Care
Cleveland, Ohio 1971

176 WEGNER, P.: The Vienna Definition Language
ACM Computing Surveys 4 (1972), 5-63

177 WELIN, C.W.: Semantic Networks and Natural Language Understanding
In: [144], 19-28

178 WINGERT, F.: Medical Language Data Processing
In: [133], 579-646

179 WINGERT, F.: Morphosyntactical Analysis of Medical Compound Word Forms
In: [144], 79-89

180 WINGERT, F.: PAULA: Programm zur Auswertung logischer Ausdrücke
Meth. Inform. Med. 11 (1972), 96-103

181 WINGERT, F.: Word Segmentation and Morpheme Dictionary for Pathology Data Processing
In: [7], 915-921

182 WINGERT, F. (Edt.): Klartextverarbeitung
Berlin, Heidelberg, New York 1978

183 WINGERT, F., GRÄPEL, P.: Systematized Nomenclature of Pathology. Deutsche Übersetzung
Schriftenreihe des Instituts für Medizinische Informatik und Biomathematik der Univ. Münster, Heft 1, 1975

184 WINGERT, F., RIES, P.: Pathologie-Befund-System
Meth. Inform. Med. 12 (1973), 150-155

185 WINKLER, C., KNOPP, R.: DV-Systeme für klinische Nuklearmedizin
In: [143], 150-162

186 WINSTON, P.H.: Artificial Intelligence
London 1977

187 WITTIG, T.: Semantische Analyse von Sätzen zur Erfassung eines Sachverhaltes
Inaug. Diss., Hamburg 1976

188 WOLFF-TERROINE, M.: CANCERNET (SABIR): An European Network for Cancer Literature
In: [150], 301-305

189 WOODS, W.A.: Transition Network Grammars for Natural Language Analysis
CACM 13 (1970), 591-606

190 WORLD HEALTH ORGANIZATION: WHO Report on Consultation on Standardization of Hospital-Based Cancer Registries
Can/73 3. Geneva 1972

191 YOUNG, D.W.: Assessment of Questions and Questionaries
Meth. Inform. Med. 10 (1971), 222-228

192 YOUNG, T.Y., CALVERT, T.W.: Classification, Estimation and Pattern Recognition
New York, London, Amsterdam 1974

193 ZYWIETZ, C.: Das EKG-System an der Medizinischen Hochschule Hannover und die Möglichkeiten eines wirtschaftlichen Einsatzes der computerunterstützten EKG-Auswertung
In: [143], 70-82

8. Index of Tables

9. Index of Figures

10. Glossary

The medical terms are partially explained following [131].

Adenocarcinoma: Particular form of a carcinoma*.

Angiography: Roentgenologic presentation of vessels after administration of a contrast medium.

Aphakia: Absence of lens (eye).

Appendectomy: Surgical removal of appendix.

Appendicitis: Inflammation of appendix.

Arachnoidea: Part of meninges.

Auscultation: Diagnosis of sounds generated in the body (heart, lungs, intestine).

Blood pressure, diastolic: Minimal arterial blood pressure during diastole of the heart.

Blood pressure, systolic: Maximal arterial blood pressure during systole of the heart.

Bronchitis: Inflammation of bronchus.

Carcinoid: Semimalignant tumor ("similar to carcinoma").

Carcinoma: Malignant epithelial tumor.

Carcinoma simplex: Special form of a carcinoma*.

Carcinosis: In an organ or the whole body localized multiple metastases* of a carcinoma*.

Cephalosporin: Antibiotic drug, similar to penicillin.

Certain event: Event occurring with probability 1.

Coelom: Fetal body cavity formed from mesoderm.

Colitis ulcerosa: Special form of an inflammation of the colon*.

Colon: Large intestine.

Complete system: System of sets decomposing* a given set.

Corpus luteum: Yellow body.

Corticoid: Corticosteroid hormone.

Craniotomy: Opening of the skull.

Cytostatic drug: Substance for inhibition of cell growth or reproduction.

Decomposition: Complete break down of a set into a set of pairwise disjoint* subsets.

Defect of aortic value: Narrowing or incomplete closure of aortic valve.

Differential blood count: Distribution of cells determined in a stained blood smear.

DIN: German standard.

Disjoint: Sets without common elements.

Diuretic drug: Drug stimulating urine flow.

Dura mater: Part of the meninges.

Dyspnea: Difficulty in breathing.

ECG: Electrocardiography, recording the variations of the electric potentials of the heart.

E. coli: Bacterium belonging to the normal intestinal flora (E.=Escherichia).

EDP: Electronic data processing.

EEG: Electroencephalography, recording the variations of the electric potentials of the brain.

Electrocardiogram: ECG*.

Electroencephalogram: EEG*.

Electromyogram: EMG*.

Electroretinogram: ERG*.

EMG: Electromyogram, recording the electric potentials of musculary actions.

ERG: Electroretinogram, recording the electric potentials of the retina.

ESR: Erythrocyte sedimentation rate.

Expectation (value): Sum of the products of possible results and probabilities of a random variable.

Geriatry: Medical science of aging.

Glomerulitis: Inflammation of a glomerulus*.

Glomerulus: Spheric structure in the kidney containing blood vessels and tubules.

Glycosuria: Excretion of glucose in urine.

Granulosaephithelioma: Tumor of granulose cells.

Hardware: Computer equipment - see software.

Heart murmor: Pathologic sound phenomenon in auscultation* of the heart.

Hemorrhage: Bleeding.

Hypalbuminemia: Decreased concentration of albumin in blood.

Hyperglycemia: Increased concentration of glucose in blood.

Hypertension: High blood pressure.

Hypertension, renal: Hypertension* caused by a disease of the kidney.

Hypertension, renovascular: Hypertension* caused by a disease of the kidney artery.

Icterus neonatorum: Jaundice of the newborn.

Incidence: Ratio of new cases of a given disease in a specified population.

Indicator variable: Random variable with the values 0 or 1.

Kidney pelvis: Cavity in the kidney for collection of urine drained by the ureters.

Labyrinth: Inner ear.

Laryngectomy: Removal of the voice box.

Laryngotracheobronchitis: Inflammation of larynx*, trachea* and bronchus.

Larynx: Voice box.

Linitis plastica: Special form of a carcinoma* of the stomach.

Metastasis: Transmission of a disease from one place to another within the body.

Morbus Hodgkin: Tumor-like proliferation of the reticulo-endothelial system*.

Myogenous: Generated in muscles.

Myopia: Shortsightedness.

Necrosis: Death of tissue.

Neoplasm: Tumor.

Nephritis: Inflammation of the kidney.

Nephrosis: Degenerative disease of the kidney.

Neurogenous: Generated in nerve (system).

Oncology: Science of real tumors.

Ophthalmology: Science of eye diseases.

Pachymeninx: Dura mater*.

Palpation: Examination by touch.

Paroxysmal: Sudden, intense attack.

Pathogenesis: Development of pathologic alterations (in contrast to cause: etiology).

Pelvic kidney: Displacement of kidney in the pelvis.

Percussion: Examination by sound.

Peritonitis: Inflammation of the peritoneum.

Phonocardiogram: Recording of heart sounds.

Plasma cell myeloma: Systemic disease with malignant proliferation of plasma cells.

Pneumencephalography: Roentgenologic examination of the (cerebral) ventricles after filling with air.

Polyarthritis: Inflammation occurring in several joints.

Probability distribution: System of probabilities for a set of events. Mathematically usually described by the distribution function or by the density (function) of a random variable.

Prostaglandin: Hormone-like substance.

Pyelonephritis: Inflammation of the kidney pelvis*.

Reticulo-endothelial system: Diffuse organ comprising all phagocytes except leucocytes.

RNA: Ribonucleic acid.

RR: Measuring arterial blood pressure by use of a Riva-Rocci sphygmomanometer.

Software: Computer programs - see Hardware.

Trachea: Bronchial tube.

Tracheitis: Inflammation of the trachea*.

Tracheobronchitis: Inflammation of the trachea* and of the bronchus.

Ulcus ventriculi: Ulcer in the stomach.

Uremia: Clinical syndrome caused by retention of substances usually excreted in the kidney.

Urogenital system: System of urinary and sexual organs.

VCG: Vectorcardiography, recording of the orthogonal leads in ECG*.

11. Symbols and Denotations

$a < b$	a is less than b
$a \leq b$	a is less than or equal to b
$a > b$	a is greater than b
$a \geq b$	a is greater than or equal to b
ld	logarithm with base 2 (ld $n \simeq 3.32 \cdot {}_{10}\log n$)
∞	sign of infinity
$(a,b]$	left open, right closed interval
$:=$	equal per definition
$\triangleq$	corresponds to
$x = \begin{cases} a, & B_1 \\ b, & B_2 \end{cases}$	x receives value a, if condition B_1 is fulfilled, or value b, if condition B_2 is fulfilled
$\sum$	summation symbol
$\sum_{i \neq j}$	Sum on all (possible) i, which are not equal to j
$k!$	factorial k
$\rightleftharpoons$	if and only if
$\lceil r \rceil$	smallest integer k with $k \geq r$
$\lfloor r \rfloor$	largest integer k with $k \leq r$
$\lvert r \rvert$, $\lvert \beta \rvert$	absolute value of number r or vector β
$\simeq$	approximately equal to
$\neq$	not equal to
a modulo b	remainder in division of the integer a by the integer b
$x = \begin{cases} a, & B \\ b, & \text{otherwise} \end{cases}$	x receives value a, if condition B is fulfilled; otherwise x receives value b

Set theory

$\{\ldots\}$	set of elements
$a \in A$	a is element of A
$\bar{A}$	complement of A
$\emptyset$	empty set
$A \subseteq B$	A is subset of B
$A \nsubseteq B$	A is not subset of B
$A \supseteq B$	A is superset of B
$A \cup B$	union of A and B
$A \cap B$	intersection of A and B

Logics

$a \wedge b$	a and b
$a \vee b$	a or b
$\bar{a}$	not a
$a \rightarrow b$	if a, then b

Statistics

$P(A)$	probability of A
$P(A \mid B)$	probability of A given B
$E(X)$	expectation of X
$\bar{x}$	(arithmetic) mean
$\tilde{x}$	empirical median
x_i	i-th date for the attribute X
x_i^*	i-th level of attribute X
μ	expectation (value)
$\tilde{\mu}$	median
σ^2	variance
χ_f^2	chi-square distribution with f degrees of freedom
$N(\mu, \sigma^2)$	normal distribution with expectation μ and variance σ^2
$x_{.j}$	$\sum_i x_{ij}$
$x_{i.}$	$\sum_j x_{ij}$

Formal languages

$a \rightarrow b$	a can be substituted by b
$a \rightarrow b \mid c$	a can be substituted by b or c
ϵ	null string

12. Subject Index

Lecture Notes in Medical Informatics

Vol. 1: Medical Informatics Europe 78. Proceedings 1978. Edited by J. Anderson. XI, 822 pages. 1978.

Vol. 2: D. Fenna, S. Abrahamsson, S. O. Lööw and H. Peterson, The Stockholm County Medical Information System. VI, 163 pages. 1978.

Vol. 3: Long-Term Studies on Side-Effects of Contraception – State and Planning. Symposium 1977. Edited by U. Kellhammer and K. Überla. VI, 240 pages. 1978.

Vol. 4: Clinical Trials in 'Early' Breast Cancer. Proceedings 1978. Edited by H. R. Scheurlen, G. Weckesser and I. Armbruster. VI, 283 pages. 1979.

Vol. 5: Medical Informatics Berlin 1979. Proceedings 1979. Edited by B. Barber, F. Grémy, K. Überla and G. Wagner. XXIII, 970 pages. 1979.

Vol. 6: Health Care Technology Evaluation. Proceedings, 1978. Edited by J. Goldman. VII, 118 pages. 1979.

Vol. 7: Technology and Health: Man and his World. Proceedings, 1978. Edited by G. Wagner, P. L. Reichertz and E. Masè. VI, 243 pages. 1980.

Vol. 8: Mathematical Aspects of Computerized Tomography. Proceedings 1980. Edited by F. Natterer. VIII, 309 pages. 1981.

Vol. 9: Computers and Mathematical Models in Medicine. Proceedings, 1977. Edited by D. Cardús and C. Vallbona. VIII, 315 pages. 1981.

Vol. 10: B. Fries, Applications of Operations Research to Health Care Delivery Systems. V, 107 pages. 1981.

Vol. 11: Medical Informatics Europe 81. Proceedings 1981. Edited by F. Grémy, P. Degoulet, B. Barber, and R. Salamon. XXIII, 975 pages. 1981.

Vol. 12: G. Wiederhold, Databases for Health Care. VI, 75 pages. 1981.

Vol. 13: The Computer and Blood Banking. Proceedings, 1981. Edited by J. R. Möhr and A. Kluge. X, 275 pages. 1981.

Vol. 14.: F. Wingert, Medical Informatics. X, 247 pages. 1981.

Medizinische Informatik und Statistik

Band 10: Perspektiven der Gesundheitssystemforschung. Frühjahrstagung, Wuppertal, 1978. Herausgegeben von W. van Eimeren. V, 171 Seiten. 1978.

Band 11: U. Feldmann, Wachstumskinetik. Mathematische Modelle und Methoden zur Analyse altersabhängiger populationskinetischer Prozesse. VIII, 137 Seiten. 1979.

Band 12: Juristische Probleme der Datenverarbeitung in der Medizin. GMDS/GRVI Datenschutz-Workshop 1979. Herausgegeben von W. Kilian und A. J. Porth. VIII, 167 Seiten. 1979.

Band 13: S. Biefang, W. Köpcke und M. A. Schreiber, Manual für die Planung und Durchführung von Therapiestudien. IV, 92 Seiten. 1979.

Band 14: Datenpräsentation. Frühjahrstagung, Heidelberg 1979. Herausgegeben von J. R. Möhr und C. O. Köhler. XVI, 318 Seiten. 1979.

Band 15: Probleme einer systematischen Früherkennung. 6. Frühjahrstagung, Heidelberg 1979. Herausgegeben von W. van Eimeren und A. Neiß. VI, 176 Seiten, 1979.

Band 16: Informationsverarbeitung in der Medizin -Wege und Irrwege-. Herausgegeben von C. Th. Ehlers und R. Klar. XI, 796 Seiten. 1980.

Band 17: Biometrie – heute und morgen. Interregionales Biometrisches Kolloquium 1980. Herausgegeben von W. Köpcke und K. Überla. X, 369 Seiten. 1980.

Band 18: R. Fischer, Automatische Schreibfehlerkorrektur in Texten. Anwendung auf ein medizinisches Lexikon. X, 89 Seiten. 1980.

Band 19: H. J. Rath, Peristaltische Strömungen. VIII, 119 Seiten. 1980.

Band 20: Robuste Verfahren. 25. Biometrisches Kolloquium der Deutschen Region der Internationalen Biometrischen Gesellschaft, Bad Nauheim, März 1979. Herausgegeben von H. Nowak und R. Zentgraf. V, 121 Seiten. 1980.

Band 21: Betriebsärztliche Informationssysteme. Frühjahrstagung, München, 1980. Herausgegeben von J. R. Möhr und C. O. Köhler. XI, 183 Seiten. 1980.

Band 22: Modelle in der Medizin. Theorie und Praxis. Herausgegeben von H. J. Jesdinsky und V. Weidtman. XIX, 786 Seiten. 1980.

Band 23: Th. Kriedel, Effizienzanalysen von Gesundheitsprojekten. Diskussion und Anwendung auf Epilepsieambulanzen. XI, 287 Seiten. 1980.

Band 24: G. K. Wolf, Klinische Forschung mittels verteilungsunabhängiger Methoden. X, 141 Seiten. 1980.

Band 25: Ausbildung in Medizinischer Dokumentation, Statistik und Datenverarbeitung. Herausgegeben von W. Gaus. X, 122 Seiten. 1980.

Band 26: Explorative Datenanalyse. Frühjahrstagung, München, 1980. Herausgegeben von N. Victor, W. Lehmacher und W. van Eimeren. V, 211 Seiten. 1980.

Band 27: Systeme und Signalverarbeitung in der Nuklearmedizin. Proceedings. Herausgegeben von S. J. Pöppl und D. P. Pretschner. IX, 317 Seiten. 1981.

Band 28: Nachsorge und Krankheitsverlaufsanalyse. 25. Jahrestagung der GMDS, Erlangen, September 1980. Herausgegeben von L. Horbach und C. Duhme. XII, 697 Seiten. 1981.

Band 29: Datenquellen für Sozialmedizin und Epidemiologie. Herausgegeben von Ralph Brennecke, Eberhard Greiser, Helmut A. Paul und Elisabeth Schach. VIII, 277 Seiten. 1981.

MIX
Papier aus verantwortungsvollen Quellen
Paper from responsible sources
FSC® C105338

If you have any concerns about our products,
you can contact us on
ProductSafety@springernature.com

In case Publisher is established outside the EU,
the EU authorized representative is:
Springer Nature Customer Service Center GmbH
Europaplatz 3, 69115 Heidelberg, Germany

Printed by Libri Plureos GmbH
in Hamburg, Germany